Foot and Mouth
Heart and Soul

A collection of personal accounts
of the foot and mouth outbreak
in Cumbria 2001

First published 2001

Text © contributors
Selection © Caz Graham
Cartoons © Colin Shelbourn, www.shelbourn.com
reproduced by kind permission of The Westmorland Gazette
Photographs © John Darwell, George Studholme, News & Star,
Keswick Reminder, Farm Stock Photography, National Trust,
Daily Telegraph, Expo Life and with kind permission of contributors.
David Maclean's article was first published in the 'House Magazine',
22nd March 2001.

Cover Picture © Jean Roper of Penruddock, Penrith

The articles in this book are personal recollections of the foot and mouth outbreak and do not reflect the views of the BBC.

Published by Small Sister for BBC Radio Cumbria

BBC Radio Cumbria,
Annetwell Street,
Carlisle,
Cumbria.
CA3 8BB

Tel: 01228 592444
www.bbc.co.uk/radiocumbria

ISBN No. 0-9541547-0-3

Printed by Sadlers, Wigton, Cumbria CA7 9SJ

Acknowledgements
Caz Graham wishes to thank all of the contributors to this book who made time to write down their thoughts and feelings. For some this involved reliving painful experiences and revisiting difficult events and raw emotions. Thank you.

Thanks also to Cumbria County Council, The Lake District National Park Authority, The National Trust, Nigel Dyson, Keith Sutton, Colin Shelbourn, Rigby Jerram, Julie Stebbings, Helen Hutchinson, Jenny de Robeck, Phil and Graham Sadler, Fiona Mills and the many other people who have offered invaluable help and advice.

Contents

Into the Valleys of Death by Peter Frost-Pennington   7

Peter Frost-Pennington	Vet	9
Gordon Swindlehurst	BBC Radio Cumbria	13
Nick Utting	NFU	15
Gordon Savage	Farmer	18
George Studholme	Slaughter man	21
Eric Worsley	Hotel Consultant	24
Rhoda Tyson	Watendlath cafe proprietor	28
Chris Bonington	Mountaineer	32
Margaret Buckle	Farmer	34
Lord Inglewood	MEP	48
Gordon Routledge	Local historian, Longtown	50
David Maclean	MP	53
Anne Hopper	BBC Radio Cumbria	58
Maggie Norton	Writer	62
Sarah Beattie	Schoolgirl	64
Marje Thomlinson	Caldew School	65
June Terry	Blindcrake resident	71
Trevor Hebdon	Harrison and Hetherington Ltd	74
Jenny de Robeck	Sebergham resident	77
Brigadier Alex Birtwistle	Retired Army officer	80
Pauline Smith	Wiggonby resident	92
Margaret Redmond & Jacqui Spanton	Ireby and Uldale residents	103
Dr Jim Cox	GP	105
Heidi Jackson	Farmer's daughter	108

Debbie Steele	Cumbria Stress Info. Network	110
Marie Stockdale	Farmer	112
Caz Graham	BBC	118
John Darwell	Photographer	125
Colin Shelbourn	Cartoonist	131
Hunter Davies	Writer	133
John Malone	Fell access point attendant	136
Deborah Cowin	Cumbria Crisis Alliance	141
Martin Rushton	Hotelier	145
John Collier	Riding school proprietor	149
Stewart Young	Cumbria County Council	153
Andrew Beeforth	Cumbria Community Recovery Fund	156
Valerie Edmondson	Lake District National Park ranger	160
Oliver Maurice	The National Trust	166
Russell Bowman	BBC Radio Cumbria diarist	170
Allan Miller	Fell runner	173
Anne Gallagher	Hawkshead Village Fair	175
Holly the Collie	Redundant sheepdog	179
Mary Forster	Farmer	181
John Graham	Farmer	184
Rev. David Wood	Priest	186
Nick Green	Heart of Cumbria	189
Andrew Humphries	Council for Agriculture and Rural Life	192
Pamela Brough	Writer	195
Les Armstrong	NFU	198
Martin Lewes	BBC Radio Cumbria	201

Foot and Mouth – Heart and Soul

It seems absurd. Here we are in the 21st century; surgeons in the States can sit at computer terminals and perform life saving operations on patients on the other side of the world. Mountaineers on Everest can find their exact location thanks to global positioning systems. We've even cracked the human genome. Yet in a matter of months a microscopic organism, a thousand times smaller than a pinhead, can still wreak untold havoc on the lives of many thousands of people in the developed world. It's humbling, a reminder of our human fallibility.

The foot and mouth virus caused billions of pounds worth of damage to the economy, not to mention the emotional scars that will mark some people for the rest of their lives.

Cumbria was hard hit. Harder hit than any other part of the UK. The virus swept through the north of the county like a tornado, swallowing everything in its path, leaving a smoky trail of misery, disbelief and devastation. Neighbours of the afflicted barricaded themselves in and gazed on in trepidation through a haze of disinfectant, doing all they could to stop such brutal violation of their own farmsteads. At times it seemed there would be no livestock left standing between Shap and Moffat. Then came the ripple effect. Except the ripples were more like tidal waves, leaving in their wake a tourist drought, empty hotels, lay-offs, and a rural economy straining under new and unprecedented pressures.

BBC Radio Cumbria broadcast from the heart of the crisis. We were relied on for fast and accurate reporting of the facts, our ability to understand and capture the mood of the community, and our regular scrutiny of key decision makers. Our news teams worked flat out on every aspect of the disease and its effect on every part of the Cumbrian community. We introduced a five-minute foot and mouth bulletin that ran seven times a day at the peak of the outbreak. Anne Hopper writes later in this book of her experiences compiling and presenting it. We broadcast a two-hour nightly phone-in to cope with the huge outpouring of public outrage and private grief. It was called Nightline and I presented and produced it. The programme ran for a month and without fail had more callers than it could cope with.

Night after night there were stories of real heartache, huge frustration and often complete fury at, and incomprehension of, the strategies and procedures that were supposed to be stopping the spread of the virus. Voices crackled down the phone lines, strained with anger, frustration and barely concealed emotion. Like many of my colleagues I would sometimes sit on the other side of the microphone with tears pricking the corners of my eyes, shaking my head at the hopelessness of it all. Reporting on foot and mouth for me, and many others, became all consuming.

Normally I like the impermanence of radio, its catch it or miss it, here today, gone tomorrow nature, never to be repeated, always making way for something new. But this was different. It felt wrong that all of the anger, the frustration, the apparent injustices should be lost into the ether each night. It seemed to me that these voices, these testimonies, needed to be recorded more permanently. So I set about doing this.

The result is this collection of writing. These are personal accounts of the foot and mouth outbreak, a sort of *written* radio programme, if you like. Most of the contributors were asked to write down their thoughts. Others provided text they'd already scribbled down, often in the wee small hours, often when there seemed nowhere else to offload pent-up emotions. You may not agree with some of the opinions voiced here. You may feel that some of these recollections don't portray events as you remember them, or in a way that rings true for you. But every account here embodies the reality of foot and mouth for people who found their lives caught up in its trail. They are here to give a flavour of how foot and mouth took root in Cumbria and touched so many lives, often the lives of people who would never have imagined that an ancient virus affecting cloven-footed animals could have anything to do with life in 21st century Britain.

The collection of writing was compiled in August, but many of the diary entries were written long before that. 'Into the Valleys of Death' on the facing page was written by Peter Frost-Pennington who was working as a Temporary Veterinary Inspector for MAFF. It caused a huge reaction when it was read on BBC Radio Cumbria and it seems a fitting way to begin to tell the story of foot and mouth in our county, the story of Cumbria in 2001.

Caz Graham
September 2001

Into The Valleys Of Death

Damien Hurst has nothing on me.
I create ghastly pictures of death, officially sanctioned.

I have to believe this mass sacrifice of animals I love
Is worth it.
Or is it the farmers who are the real sacrifice?
Like the animals, they take it meekly and obediently
Often thanking me for doing it.
After I had killed all 356 cattle in one family's dairy herd
They sent flowers to my wife.
These are the people who are giving up all, in the hope it will save others.

But don't get me wrong
I have now seen plenty of this plague
And it is no common cold.
The animals suffer horribly, as the skin of their tongues peels off
And their feet fall apart.
We must try to kill them quick and clean,
As soon as it appears in a herd or flock.

The farmers' suffering does not end with the visit of the
Slaughter men.

I must continue to do my duty
In these Cumbrian killing fields.
Quickly, efficiently and effectively.
Yes, the official papers must all be in place
Yes, the Health and Safety Man must be happy
Yes, the Environment Agency are only doing their job as best they can.

It is 6 a.m. Today I go out to kill again.
The worst is the young stock.
I thank God the lambs are not yet born with these ewes today.
I will have to kill a calf born yesterday,
The first beautiful calf from the farmer's pride and joy
His new Charolais bull.

This is not what I trained for.
I hope familiarity will never make me immune from the trauma of killing
But I do hope – for the animals' sake – to be good at it.

It is the virus we are trying to kill
With our disinfectants and culling policy
Our imprisonment of farmers in their own homes
All they have left is the telephone.

Perhaps today there is hope
One soldier will meet me at the farm gate
I hope he, not me, will quickly arrange the funeral of the animals I
    love
Before their carcasses get so bloated they fall apart
Adding more to the farmer's anguish, trapped amongst them.
I should be free to move on quickly, find the virus
And kill again.

Into the Valleys of Death drove the 600
Or are we now 1100?
The countryside I love is bleeding to death
Mr Blair, please help.

Peter Frost-Pennington
Temporary Veterinary Inspector
23rd March 2001

Peter Frost-Pennington

Peter Frost-Pennington wrote 'Into the Valleys of Death' *while working as a Temporary Veterinary Inspector for the Ministry of Agriculture, Fisheries and Food during the early days of the foot and mouth outbreak. The poem seemed to express the despair, hopelessness and impotence that so many people felt at that time. Hundreds of listeners wrote to BBC Radio Cumbria for copies and Peter was invited to recite it at the Royal Albert Hall before the Prince of Wales to raise money for farming charities. A qualified vet by profession, Peter has spent the last ten years working in the tourism industry, renovating and helping run Muncaster Castle near Ravenglass.*

The Silent Spring

Words can never express the depths of people's feelings in those dark days of spring 2001. Foot and mouth disease, the most virulent virus known to mankind, stalked our beloved countryside. Although non-infectious to humans, my goodness how it affects us! This ghastly pestilence suddenly erupted in the four corners of England and didn't spare Wales, Scotland or Ireland either, but the biggest weight of infection was in Cumbria. In early March, the State Veterinary Service simply had not enough of anything, especially vets, and the terrible virus was running days ahead of us. It was horrible to see how quickly this unseen monster could devastate and cause huge suffering to herds and flocks of cloven-hoofed animals. Killing these beautiful animals as fast as we could was the only weapon we were allowed to use.

Since the virus is shed in large quantities *before* the infected animal shows any signs, we had to kill many animals who appeared to be perfectly healthy as we got on with our gruesome task as best we could. This is a huge quandary for many people, particularly vets, as few people object to animals being 'put out of their misery', but to kill them before they are 'miserable' is hard to bear. And yet, without doing that, these apparently 'healthy' animals can act like factories, shedding huge quantities of this virus into the environment. This means more animals suffer, and more livelihoods are destroyed.

It was not only the blood, the tears, the mud, the acrid plumes of smoke or the stench of rotting carcasses. It was also the silence. The imprisonment. The lack of information. The frustration and hopelessness. The fear. The waiting.

The biggest tragedy of the whole disaster is how the disease has torn communities apart. Neighbour has been set against neighbour. Normal activities have been erased from the calendar. Rumour pervades the air like the plumes from the funeral pyres and, like the virus itself, rumours also spread like wildfire. Everyone wants somebody else to blame, and a whole vicious circle of claim and counter claim feeds on itself developing suspicion, mistrust and enmity.

Immersed in the most soul-destroying job I have ever been asked to do, I have been amazed by the fortitude, courage, friendliness, kindness and strength of spirit I have been privileged to see in the most resilient group of people I know - farmers. Strong and passionate about their animals and the bare earth they farm, this year I have seen many cry. I have also seen many shout and wail out in anger. Although I have been on the receiving end of their pent-up frustration and fury, it has never been directed at me, but at the draconian and sometimes incomprehensible 'system' that has been imposed on them to try and kill off the disease, but we must remember it is this tiny organism that has devastated and affected so many lives. Nor is it just the farmers; so many people have suffered as a result of this plague. Before volunteering as one of the first 'Temporary Veterinary Inspectors' to help fight the disease, I had spent the previous few years working full-time helping to run a major tourist attraction, so I know also the calamity it has caused to this large and important industry. There can be, however, few

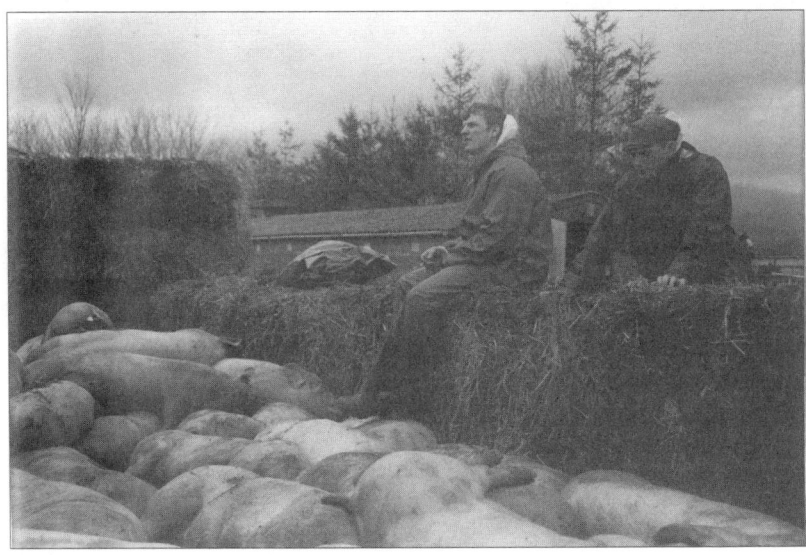

Photo: George Studholme

tortures worse than, within a single day, watching all those cherished animals you have spent years of your life breeding, rearing and protecting from harm, killed in front of your eyes. In many cases, you offer cups of tea and scones to those involved, and say 'thank you' as they leave you alone on your silent, dead farm.

It was this raw emotion and passion, combined with frustration and desperation that caused me to have one of many sleepless nights in March 2001. I still do not really believe I composed my poem – it simply tumbled onto the page early in the morning of 23rd March 2001, and after little more than 20 minutes was finished. I did not know why I had written it, except I suppose, as a plea for help. I faxed it in a raw, handwritten scrawl to my wife Iona before rushing out to destroy yet another farm, including a proud, huge bull and a tiny and beautiful day-old calf – his first offspring. I think I telephoned Iona and asked if it could be sent, perhaps as a letter to the papers, in the hope it could make people who were looking on with complacent, uncaring eyes, a little more appreciative of what farmers, vets, and many others involved with the whole ghastly process, were going through.

I never could have imagined the response to my 'emotional outburst'. My father-in-law, Patrick Gordon Duff Pennington, a farmer himself and long a champion of their battles, rang up BBC Radio Cumbria and read it to them. They liked it, and recorded it. They played it early one morning, as a 'one-off' and the telephone lit up like a Christmas tree. People requested it again and again – it was played on the radio many times. So many asked for a copy, they put it on their web site. Still working hard, I was only peripherally aware of the response, and it was a week or more before I saw a written copy of the poem and realised there were two minor mistakes – my father-in-law had difficulty reading my handwritten fax! I was invited to Radio Cumbria and read the poem myself.

To say it snowballed is an understatement. And so it was that, on the evening of 18th April 2001, I found myself all alone on the stage of the Royal Albert Hall in London, with 5,000 people watching from the darkness, including the Prince of Wales. The Farm Aid concert, conceived and organised within a month, had included readings from such poets as Rupert Brooke, Robert Graves and William Wordsworth, as well as a heart-rending account by a Berkshire pig farmer of the trauma of watching his life's work being slaughtered. Mine was the penultimate act. Standing centre stage, heart pounding, I recited my poem to total silence. Not one pin was heard to drop, until a wave of applause filled the void. The retiring collection took £35,000, and I hope my recital squeezed an extra pound or two into the buckets. The concert raised £365,000 for agricultural charities, and it was hugely humbling to be a part of it.

Now set to music by local composer John Lipscombe, and released on a CD, sales and direct donations for a copy of the poem have to date directly raised over £1,500. This is a tiny drop in an ocean of suffering, but it seems my words encapsulated some of the emotions of those early and very dark days. At the time of writing this piece, we are still struggling to control this devastating foe, and have by no means won the war, but I hope I can return to my more usual life of giving people pleasure, not pain, as they visit this most beautiful, cherished, varied yet tragic county. I hope 'Into the Valleys of Death' does capture some of the grief and anguish of the crisis, helps those who have suffered more than me and brings some understanding to those who have not.

In many cases, it is the farmers who still have their stock who are now suffering far more, having been trapped on their farms for many months with no income and many hungry mouths to feed, as well as trying their best to 'maintain good bio-security', a rather ill-defined and often misunderstood buzz phrase. The complexities of farming under the emergency restrictions frequently make life nearly impossible. Tenants in particular have seen the value of their livestock, their only collateral, reduced to a mere fraction.

The last two words of my poem are just as relevant as I write now in August, as they were in March 2001. I fear they will be relevant for months and years to come... 'Please help.'

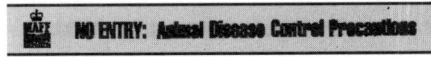

Gordon Swindlehurst

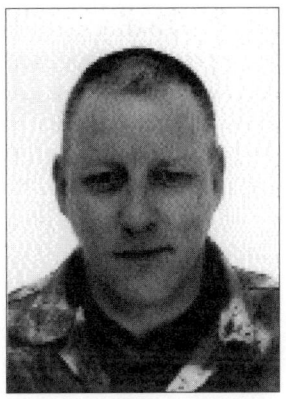

The BBC journalist Gordon Swindlehurst was working in Birmingham as a producer on Radio 4's flagship agriculture programme, Farming Today, when foot and mouth was discovered in Britain. He subsequently returned to cover the crisis in Cumbria as the county became the area worst affected by the disease. Here he recalls a day he will never forget: Tuesday, February 20th, 2001.

Even without a mirror, I could tell the colour had drained from my face. What we'd feared all afternoon had finally been confirmed. Foot and mouth had been discovered at an abattoir in Essex. And that was bad news for British agriculture - and worse still for Cumbria.

The initial call from the ministry had come around lunchtime. They thought they'd detected the disease in pigs at Brentwood - the Meat and Livestock Commission was more upbeat: 'We think it'll prove negative,' said a spokesman. But a few, short hours later, the call came through: 'Confirmed.'

We hotfooted it back to the studio to turn the next day's farming programme on its head. There was a new interview with the minister, but my piece on what foot and mouth is, cribbed from the infant recess of the brain and Black's veterinary dictionary, stayed as it was.

So too the item with a former chairman of the farmers' union in Worcester, looking back to the dark days of disinfectant and quicklime in 1967. That had been commissioned a few weeks earlier, when the Government banned live imports from South Africa because of foot and mouth there. Even in mid-January, before anyone suspected the plague would be upon us, before winter had pulled in its claws, those three little words had had a galvanising effect.

My earliest memory of childhood was of my brother coming home from milking, the sweet scent of cows on his clothes swamped by the acrid stench of chemicals. For years thereafter, the mere mention of the disease brought sickness to men's stomachs and a panic to their eyes - the panic I felt on my own face on the evening of February 20th.

A dread disease the industry had thought was gone forever was back in the country. In the thirty-odd years since that last big outbreak, British farming had changed, almost beyond recognition. It had fallen into new ways of working, without ever shaking off the wartime credo that farmers had a duty to us all to produce as much food as they could, as cheaply as possible. And so the fields and farm buildings of Cumbria were crammed with cattle and sheep. But it wasn't the sheer weight of animals which boded black. One of the developments of the decades had been the growth of the county as a strategic centre for British livestock. A mere glance at the map shows Carlisle close to the geographical dead centre of these islands. It's a point hammered home in visits to rural communities throughout the land. So many people I'd met throughout the nation in six months at Farming Today had told me: 'Yes, we come to Carlisle for our cattle and Longtown for our sheep.'

And it was this which made the Cumbrian catastrophe inevitable. Not just the method of farming, nor the reputation of this corner of England as a provider of pedigree breeds and quality meat, but its magnetic attraction for traders the length and breadth of Britain.

I'm sure there were friends who wondered why I was so distraught, that grim night in the bar at Pebble Mill. They couldn't comprehend how an animal disease they'd hardly heard of could fill a hard-headed hack with such obvious fear. They wouldn't get the tearful phone calls from proud, strong men whose cattle would be culled and lie dead outside the door for days. And they wouldn't have to live with the sense of helplessness as a way of life fell to dust. I was, and did, and will.

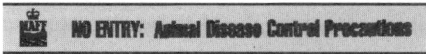

Nick Utting

As Group Secretary for the National Farmers' Union in North Cumbria, Nick Utting found himself right at the centre of the crisis from day one. He became a familiar face, regularly interviewed by local, national and international press. He was a key figure at Ministerial and Prime Ministerial visits, and found himself working seven days a week to look after his members' interests.

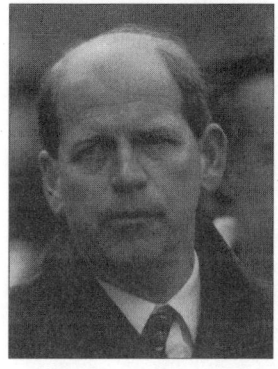

No one outside our beautiful county can truly understand the devastation caused by the terrible virus that is foot and mouth. I would not criticise outsiders for that, because even if they drove through our countryside during March and April of 2001, nature was still producing its usual array of spring beauty. Yes, there were the terrible pyres and rotting carcasses which hit the headlines, but few saw the brutal effects on the lives and inner feelings of everyone throughout the rural communities and of course particularly the farming families who experienced the disease hitting their own cherished stock.

Those of us who were lucky enough not to experience the world wars, now appreciate what 'blitz' conditions were like, but without the exploding bombs and wrecked properties. Instead of the human bodies, we had thousands and thousands of animal carcasses destroyed before our eyes and the mental anguish which engulfed us all.

This is not the time to lay blame, but much of the anguish was caused by Government's inability to operate a plan to cope with such disasters and their knee jerk decisions which affected all our lives so dramatically on a daily basis as the crisis unfolded during March and April. As local secretaries to the NFU, we were very much involved in the daily discussions with MAFF and endeavoured to represent the interests of all in north Cumbria. We had some lengthy and painful meetings.

Whilst we endeavoured to influence policy for our county, and did so on many occasions, much of the time we were forced to ponder with amazement the decisions and actions of senior civil servants and politicians. May I share with you two such occasions.

Firstly, I will relate the unbelievable devastation caused by Nick Brown, then Minister of Agriculture, when panic had set in at the rapid spread of the disease in north Cumbria. It had been mooted that the Minister was to make a lunchtime announcement regarding some form of livestock cull to halt the disease spread. Rumours were that this would involve sheep in a wide circle around the main infected area of Cumbria. All farmers in our county, and of course us as officials, were glued to our TVs and radios for the announcement.

The panic and confusion caused by the subsequent announcement were beyond belief. Not only did the Minister announce a cull of healthy sheep as a 'fire-break', but all cattle in north Cumbria were also to be slaughtered. We could not believe it, but that was exactly what was to happen and was confirmed by phone, fax and email within a matter of minutes.

We were totally shell-shocked. The phone for the next few hours went berserk and all ended up in tears at the thought of what was to happen to some of the finest herds in the country. I remember having previously been asked to attend that afternoon a meeting of the full Carlisle City Council to explain the disease situation. Somehow or other I managed to drive to the Council Chamber, but how I managed to present my report I shall never know. I can remember my voice being very shaky and one Council member passing me some water. I concluded by giving the latest devastating news and fought back the tears. This particular day concluded with a further unbelievable statement by the Minister when he clarified his earlier announcement by saying that cattle would not be culled in north Cumbria. I am afraid Mr Brown that your apology did little to help us sleep that night.

Another most remarkable day, which will remain with me for a long time to come, was the first time that Tony Blair came to Cumbria.

Things were really going wrong, in fact from bad to worse. The number of cases was increasing daily, with no signs of stopping, and of course MAFF could just not cope with the number of animals to be diagnosed with the disease, and the mounting heaps of carcasses requiring disposal. The Army had finally been brought in, but was still under the control of MAFF.

About a dozen of us sat round one table with the Prime Minister, farmers, MAFF, local authorities, businessmen, and of course Brigadier Birtwistle. All relating the same picture of backlog and devastation. All complaining about the delays being caused by Whitehall and the Government's civil servants. Having listened to our desperate stories the Prime Minister turned to his MAFF officials and gave them the authority to diagnose on clinical signs, and to the Brigadier he gave authority to write whatever cheques were necessary to remove the carcasses, by whatever means were necessary.

It was quite amazing what happened next. As the meeting concluded the Army moved into action and finally, *finally*, we started to see essential

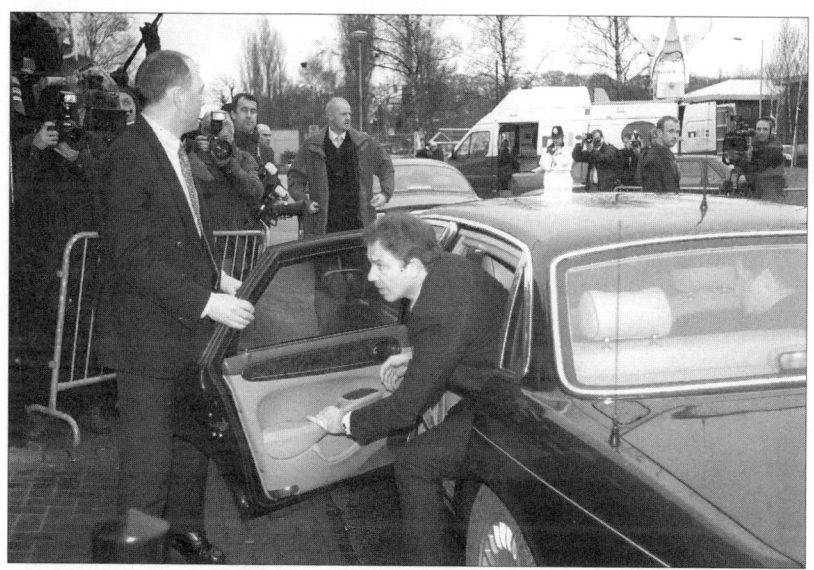

Photo: News & Star

Tony Blair arriving at Rosehill in Carlisle

measures being taken. And about time too. Many weeks later, when his personal job was done, the Brigadier was heard to say 'we are not proud of what we had to do, but we are proud of the way we did it'.

I have never been a fan of politics, and certainly the last few months have not made me any more interested. I have now learned, however, the meaning of political 'spin', which has reared its ugly head so many times throughout this terrible time for our county.

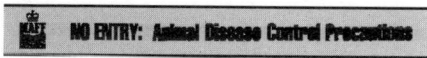

Gordon Savage

Gordon Savage farmed at Bank End Farm, Hesket Newmarket for 21 years. In 1992 the tenancy was handed over to his daughter Jane and son-in-law Geoff. This is Gordon's diary from the week the farm lost its stock to foot and mouth.

Monday 26th March 2001

......will always be known as Black Monday. The day the slaughter men arrived to destroy all the stock on Bank End Farm, leaving two dogs and two cats. We knew in our heart of hearts that it was going to happen, but when it eventually did, it was still a tremendous shock. The saying goes that 'where there is life there is hope' and you just pray for a miracle, but reality catches up and that dreadful day has dawned.

At 9 o'clock this morning cattle were mooing and lambs were bleating, already over 300 lambs had been born, ewes were looking in good condition and grass was beginning to awake from its winter sleep. It was nearly Easter with summer to look forward to. It should be a joyous time on a farm.

At 3 o'clock - nothing left except a big pile of dead stock. Even the grass was bowing its head in the cool breeze as if it was in sympathy. Life on the farm has been difficult enough in the wake of BSE. The last five years have been a struggle with Geoff having to take a part-time job driving a lorry for a cattle feed manufacturer to help with the income. This has now come to an end. Jane has created a small bed and breakfast business to supplement the cash flow, but alas, everyone has cancelled their bookings. Life suddenly has become very empty and all the care that goes into looking after stock seems pointless. The most tragic thing was a lamb which Jane had lovingly brought into the world at 9 o'clock and which was shot at 2 o'clock. Life can be very unjust at times.

Geoff and Jane have been very strong during the crisis with their main priority being to protect their two sons from the tragedy. Daniel is busy with exams at school. Will the events affect his concentration? Geoff's brother Andrew and his wife, who is actually Jane's sister Caroline, are doing all they can to help look after their two nephews until the situation has settled down. Geoff's Mum, Sylvia, is staying at the farm, helping Jane with the housework as well as being a comforting influence. Jane's Mum, Dorothy, is helping with washing and ironing and baking. Gordon, Jane's Dad, is looking into the financial side, seeing if there are any benefits that may be available. What does the future hold?

Tuesday morning dawns and everything is covered with snow with a cold wind blowing. The little dead lambs are lying next to their dead mothers, frozen solid. Life on the farm is at its lowest ebb. Geoff and Jane have hardly slept all night. They still waken at the usual 6 o'clock time, but what for? Normally by 7 o'clock Geoff has fed all the stock and inspected the sheep, Jane has fed the pet lambs, got the two boys ready for school and made the breakfast, but this morning, nothing. Lassie, Geoff's sheepdog doesn't seem to understand why there are not any sheep. She is allowed to come into the house today and get some comfort from Jane's pet sheepdog, Ben. They both know that something is wrong.

The boys, Daniel and Jacob, have both been told that all the stock has been killed. They are relieved that Lassie and Ben haven't been shot. Grandad Savage has explained to them that life will be difficult for the next few years for their Mum and Dad. They understand. They are good lads. Jacob is sure that his very own Texel ewe and her two lambs have gone to greener pastures in the sky.

Wednesday morning arrives, a bit damp, but the snow has all gone. Jane can't cry any more, she has no more tears left. Geoff seems to have lost about a stone of weight since Saturday. His 400 big bales of silage that he usually sells this time of year are unsaleable. The rent cheque has gone through the bank and he has just been notified that his council tax will be nearly £1200. Sooner or later he will have to face the bank manager to explain his cash flow. The day is spent dealing with paperwork which seems to take their mind off the pile of dead stock lying in the yard. Geoff and Jane get a special permit to visit their two sons at Uncle Andrew and Auntie Caroline's. Both lads put their arms around their Mum which brings a few more tears from Jane.

Thursday comes with more spring like weather; a lovely day for lambing, if only! Geoff and Jane couldn't sleep for the smell of dead stock so they left their own bedroom and slept in the holiday annex which is on the far side of the house. When will they take the carcasses away? Out of sight, out of mind a bit would help. Both Geoff and Jane can't face any food because of the smell. The postman leaves some sympathy letters at the farm gate today and they learn that some of their friends have got foot and mouth disease. One or two local ladies have brought Jane some flowers to brighten her day which was very thoughtful. Geoff wondering if there was any need to have bought fertiliser which is standing in the barn. It looks like they are going to miss a year farming. It will be very doubtful if he can buy stock back later on this year if forecasted prices are anything to go by. They are back to where they started nine years ago. Having worked so hard to build stock numbers up, all seems to have disappeared in a few days. Another night sleeping in the holiday annex.

Friday morning dawns – a beautiful spring morning, much better than days had been in the middle of lambing – sod's law. Tractors and trailers arrive to take the dead stock away to put on a neighbour's pyre. At least it will get rid of some of the smell, although some of it will hang round for a few days yet. Geoff's started damping everything down with disinfectant and probably wouldn't care if he never went into the buildings ever again. At least he is doing something and seems determined to make a really exceptional job of it. Is he beginning to fight back? Jane comes out in leggings and waterproofs to help. The sooner they get rid of every sign of this terrible disease the better. Daniel had an important exam today. Hope it went OK for him.

Jane's mother is busy all day preparing a special evening meal for Andrew, Caroline, Daniel and Jacob. Nobody has eaten properly all week because of the disruption. Geoff and Jane are not allowed off the farm so they can't come. Disappointing, a family meal might have cheered them up. At least they may get a better night's sleep.

Saturday morning is wild and wet. An army man turns up to give advice. Geoff has been told that he can't use the fertiliser. It has to be disinfected and left for some time. More disinfecting done, all disease should be killed by now. Geoff has an extended lunch to watch his favourite football team, Liverpool v. Manchester United, and this lifts his spirits quite a bit. It is a week now since he suspected that a sheep had foot and mouth and informed the ministry vet.

The last seven days have been an absolute nightmare for Geoff and Jane. A week that will change their lives forever. Whatever the future holds is anybody's guess. A long think will be needed to determine in which direction life will go. Whatever happens, the last week in March 2001 will remain in the minds of Geoff and Jane forever.

Jane's Mum and Dad, Gordon and Dorothy, were trying to keep their small flock of pure Texels intact so that Geoff and Jane would have something to start again with but today they have been valued and taken away to be slaughtered in the 'buffer zone' cull.
This puts the final nail in the coffin.
There is nothing more to report.

George Studholme

George Studholme from Wigton has worked as a slaughter man for the last 26 years. He spent most of spring and summer 2001 slaughtering animals on infected farms leading a team of 8 men. He is a keen amateur photographer and took pictures of some of the scenes he came across. Two of those photos are used as illustrations in this book.

February 2001 – News was breaking that foot and mouth had been confirmed in pigs at an abattoir in Essex. I don't think many people gave it a second thought. I, however, had worked with people that had worked on the 1967/68 outbreak and can remember some of my past work colleagues talking about it. What a fight it had been to contain it.

Everyone watched the news with increased interest when it was announced that infected animals had passed through Longtown Auction, the largest sheep auction in the country and we knew then the 'shit had hit the fan'. Dealers from all over the country traded at Longtown and most farmers in Cumbria and South West Scotland used the auction. We all knew it was now just a waiting game to see what would happen.

On Friday 9th March all the staff at J & D Graham, Black Brow Abattoir at Wiggonby received their envelopes telling us that because of the livestock movement ban we were now all laid off work. Everyone went home that day not knowing where to turn next, only the thought of signing on the dole.

Next day, Saturday, two slaughter teams were thrown together and we were off to Tow Law, County Durham, to carry out the slaughter on two infected farms. The following day we were out again, but in Cumbria, where we've been ever since, day in, day out, from dawn to dusk. One farm a day, sometimes two, on occasions even three, but now as the cases subside I have time to write this account as I wait for another phone call with instructions to go to another I.P. (Infected Premises).

If I had to reflect on one farm that brings back memories, it would have to be Geoff and Billy Todhunter's at Little Bampton. We arrived at the farm on Wednesday 14th March. It was a lovely spring morning and the sun was really hot. We sat around on the road outside the farm gates waiting to start. We could hear the milking machines still going as we sat talking and we could see the Todhunters working away as normal. They could see us sitting by the gate with our matching blue waterproof suits and our guns by our sides, waiting to come in. What a sight. What must they have been thinking? I bet they wished they could have milked those cows all day to delay us from coming in. Then Paul Duff, the vet in charge arrived and went in to talk to the Todhunters. He came back shortly to tell us that they were nearly finished milking and would come and let us in when they were ready. Geoff came over to the gate to let us in, his voice breaking, he said 'I know you have got a job to do but please don't let my animals suffer'. He broke down and cried with his head in his hands, we all looked at each other dumbstruck and I'm sure we all realised then how serious this disease was.

They had nearly 700 cattle on three holdings. We started with the dairy cows and the brothers stayed with us to the end. They wouldn't leave, they insisted on not abandoning them. As the day drew to a close and all the adult cattle were slaughtered it was time to go to the calf sheds. It was Billy's turn to get upset. He told us through a flood of tears he had spent his whole life in that calf shed bringing them into the world, nursing the weak ones and helping the calves get stronger. Peter Haughan, who worked for them, was a tower of strength. He put his arm around Billy and walked him off up the yard. All that hard work and we walked in the shed and it was all over in ten minutes. There was an eerie silence, all quiet. We had finished one holding. We all got washed down and disinfected, said goodnight and would see them in the morning to do the other two sites.

We turned up in the morning and Geoff and Billy were different again, everyone was having a good crack with them, we were all laughing and joking as we walked down the village to the second holding where we swiftly started the first of the 157 cattle we had to do that day. Then we had to go to a little hamlet called Studholme to finish off the last of the cattle, then we started on their sheep. Over 400 were killed in four different fields.

We then went back to the farmhouse, had a cup of tea and as we were about to go home Billy and Geoff shook all our hands and thanked us. I had a lump in my throat as Geoff shook mine, thanking me for doing a job that I'm sure none of us will ever forget.

Even now, nearly six months later, we are all still at it. The cases are slowing down but we are still busy. It works out that we get a job every other day. We've spent the last two months slaughtering in the Shap, Appleby and Kirkby Stephen areas. We can't seem to get on top of it down there, and it is slowly creeping towards North Yorkshire where they have problems of their own. As autumn gets closer I really wish this plague would end. I can tell by everyone involved in it: vets, shepherds, slaughter men, valuers, contractors, DEFRA Officials……everyone is getting weary, we're all sick and tired of it.

The sooner we get back to normal, the better, but we all know it won't be the same again. The disease has hit Cumbria so hard that it will pave the way for the government to make wholesale agricultural policy changes.

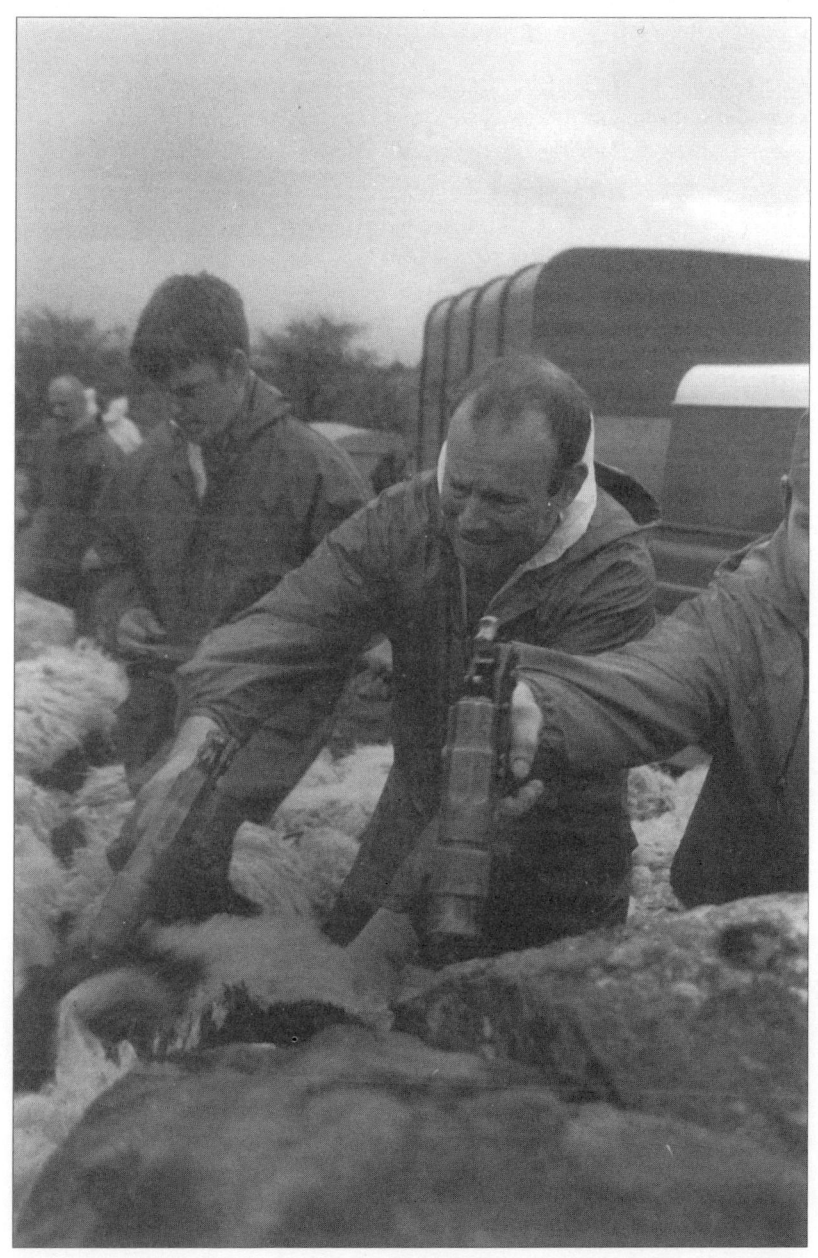

Photo: George Studholme

Eric Worsley

Eric Worsley works as an independent consultant to Lake District hoteliers. During the foot and mouth outbreak he found many of his clients severely affected by the lack of visitors to the area. He also runs a website called no-vacancies.com that became an important source of information for many hoteliers and Bed and Breakfast owners.

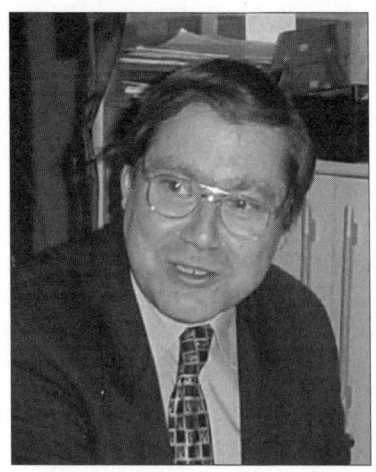

Mine is a job that city slickers dream of and country folk laugh at. I spend my working life travelling around the highways and byways of the English Lake District, visiting hotels and guest houses and advising the owners about running their business. For me, March is a very important time. It is when hotels that are closed throughout the winter come out of hibernation, and hotels that are open throughout the winter learn if it has been worthwhile.

Generally speaking, hotels don't make money in the winter, but bills still have to be paid and refurbishment carried out. So the first opportunity to make a profit is very welcome, and it is vitally important that they do make a profit in the spring, since this will offset the loss they have made during the previous months.

So for me March is a crucial period. It's either 'Yes, Mr Jones, you have had a good start to the year with lots of bookings and the situation looks rosy,' in which case they are happy, or it's, 'I'm sorry to have to tell you this, Mr Smith, but things do not look good. To put it bluntly, unless we do something now you're in big trouble.'

The fact is that no one likes to bear bad news, but when it has to be done at least I can add the sentence, 'but don't worry Mr Smith, because I've drawn up an action plan that will help you out of your predicament.' Even when a hotel is in trouble I can always point to the light at the end of the tunnel. The fact is that something can be done. Jobs can be secured, losses turned to profit, futures assured.

The winter of 2000/2001 had not been easy. 2000 was an average year until September. Then came the fuel crisis and for two weeks of what is usually the busiest month in the Lake District the roads were eerily quiet.

The fuel crisis was soon over and trade returned to normal, but the point about a hotel is that it can never recoup lost income. Unlike a shop, which can sell unsold products the following day, hotel rooms are instantly perishable. A hotel that has 10 rooms available can only sell them once each day. When that day has gone, so has the chance of selling unsold rooms.

Winter 2000 was wet and windy. Few winter tourists ventured out, but there was a feeling of optimism amongst the hotel owners of Lakeland. Generally speaking spring bookings were well up on previous years. Visitors who had stayed away the previous autumn and winter were booking in large numbers. Bookings diaries were full, the telephone was ringing and hotel owners were confident that the losses of the past six months would soon be wiped out. Then came foot and mouth.

I clearly remember the first week of March 2001. It was the worst week of my working life. I had started out in a cautious but optimistic mood. The foot and mouth crisis was gathering pace, and I knew that trade would be down but I have always believed that, barring a war, there would never be a situation where nothing could be done. The first hotel visits I made were fairly routine. Bookings had stopped coming in, but there was no great panic. What none of us involved in the tourism industry were aware of was that those in authority would effectively shut down our industry, and then announce it to the world. The closing of footpaths was expected, and we knew it would have an effect, but what was not expected was for an official of the National Park Authority to go on television and announce, 'If you don't have a reason to come the Lake District, don't!' The region's largest

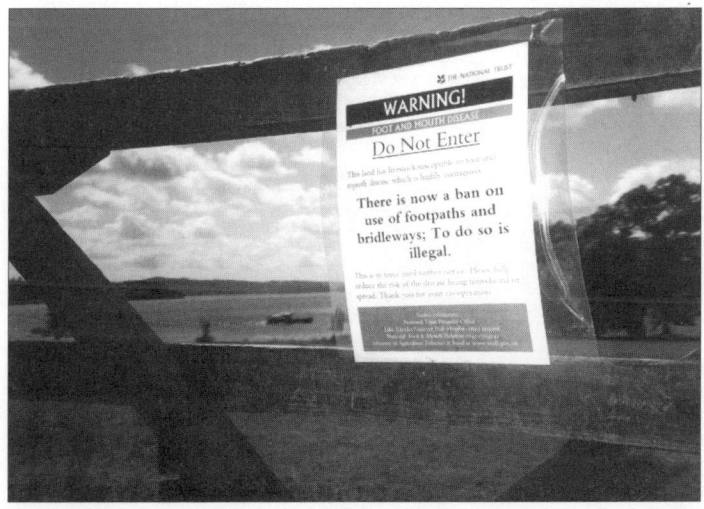

From: No-vacancies.com <hmss@no-vacancies.com>
Date: Tue, 22 May 2001 23:09:32 +0000
To: Hotels
Subject: Now you see it, now you don't

Hello Everyone

As you are no doubt aware, the Government has promised that financial aid is on the way for hard pressed businesses within Cumbria. Michael Meacher told Cumbria Crisis Alliance only a couple of weeks ago that the money had already left the treasury. But he did not know where it was. Clearly his advisors did not know either, and since Tony Blair decided to have an election all the civil servants seem to have gone off on their holidays leaving, it seems, the money to fend for itself.

The question is, if the treasury doesn't have it, where is it? I have spent much of the last 2 weeks trying to find out. I don't know the answer, but some of the mismanagement that I have uncovered during my quest beggars belief.

Two weeks ago I contacted Business Link. "Do you have the Government's money?" I asked. "Yes and No" came the reply. It seems that they have been told that they can offer local businesses 50% grants to help with marketing costs, but they don't actually have the money, and they don't know when they will get it.

"You can also get a grant towards the cost of updating your web site," they told me. They gave me the name of the man coordinating the web site grant, and told me that all I had to do was talk to him and he would sort it out. Unfortunately they did not tell him! He doesn't know anything about it. When questioned he demanded to know who had told me about him. I took the matter up with Business Link, who said that they had not told anyone that web site grants were available, and that they had not passed on anyone's name. Perhaps I dreamed it all, including the name of the coordinator and his telephone number.

The final straw with Business Link came when they told one of my clients that marketing Grants did not exist, and that he should contact Cumbria Tourist Board. Unfortunately Cumbria Tourist Board don't know anything about marketing grants, other than to offer the advice "talk to Business Link." Meanwhile another Business Link advisor told another customer of mine that Marketing grants did exist, but that they were not for 50% of marketing costs, but for 100%. She advised him to hurry before the money runs out. He replied that he had heard the money had not run in yet, so could not run out.

The fact is that Business Link do not know what is available, or when, or who they can give it to. The Government, which in effect does not exist at the moment, has not told them. It is not their (Business Links) fault. They are caught up in this mess in the same way that everyone else is, waiting for someone in Government to tell them what they can offer, and then to back it with cash!

I tried the RDA. Now they would surely have some idea of where the money is. I asked "Have you got the Governments money?" "No" they replied, "but we know who has." "Who?" I asked. "Cumbria Tourist Board," they said proudly. "Oh no they haven't" I replied. After an exchange of Pantomime proportions, they decided that I might just be right. It is not the Tourist Board after all. It is Business Link. They have the money. Or so the RDA think.

I've asked other esteemed organisations if they have the money. The National Parks Authority don't have it, The National Trust don't have it either. MAFF would like it because theirs has run out and they need some more. Cumbria County Council are staring at a £1 million shortfall in their money, and definitely have not got it. Neither have South Lakeland or any of the other District Councils. No one has the money, least of all those who need it most.

The question still remains. Where is it? Does it really exist? Whose bank is it in? Who gets the interest while it is there?

I'm going to keep looking. Because I know it is out there somewhere.........

I'll keep you posted.

Eric Worsley

no-vacancies.com

land owner, the National Trust, followed shortly afterwards. They closed down everything, regardless of whether it involved agriculture or not. The Trust shop in the middle of Hawkshead next door to the Co-op was shut and just to make sure that any stray tourists would get the message to stay away they put a sign on the door to say why it was shut. The fact is, these bodies, like the Government, carried out these acts in good faith. There was nothing malicious in their actions. They wanted to prevent foot and mouth from entering the region. As a life long member of the tourism fraternity I sat and watched as my industry was systematically shut down by people who didn't seem to realise that the medicine was doing more damage than the ailment it was intended to treat. By the middle of the first week of March the mood amongst hoteliers was far from encouraging. Cancellations were flooding in. Previously full bookings books were empty. One hotel owner told me he would be better off buying shares in Tippex than running a Lake District hotel. Then came the worst moment of the week. I made an unscheduled stop at a remote but usually busy hotel in the heart of the Lakeland fells. I had been there just a few days before, and prospects had been very good. Spring bookings were the best ever. When I entered the hotel on that Thursday lunchtime there was an eerie silence. The office, normally a hive of activity, had a solemn atmosphere. When I walked in the owner looked up, then away. He reached for a handkerchief and wiped his eyes. 'Hay fever,' he said, 'it's come early this year'. I simply agreed with him. He was a proud man. A hotel owner for a considerable number of years, always successful, always positive. I didn't want him to know that I knew he had been crying. Over the next 20 minutes I learned that he had lost £35,000 worth of forward bookings in the space of just a few hours. Which is greater than the value of all the sheep in his locality. The sheep that the shutdown policy was intended to protect. And that has been the problem. Foot and mouth disease is treated as an economic disease. Animal welfare does not come into it. If it did, we would not have murdered 2 million perfectly healthy sheep. The remedy is carried out for economic reasons, to protect the farming industry. I have no problem with that, as long as in doing so the effect on other industries is not so great that it makes grown men weep.

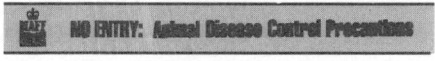

Rhoda Tyson

Rhoda Tyson runs the cafe at Watendlath, near Derwentwater. This is normally a tourist honey-pot, bustling with hungry walkers and sightseers, but for three months in March, April and May of 2001, all Rhoda sold was one Mars Bar for a princely 37p.

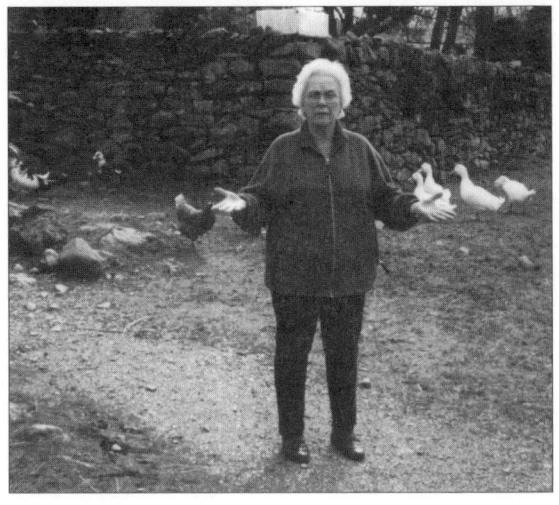

I came to Watendlath as an 18-year-old student full of enthusiasm, energy and optimism for the future. I was born and brought up in West Cumbria, the Lake District in sight of my home. At this time in my life, when I was about to start teacher training, the way ahead looked bright. The idea of coming to this remote hamlet was to earn money to subsidise a student grant. I had opted to work in the area for a month before studies began. The work in the farmhouse was non-stop and from the crack of dawn. It involved cleaning, scrubbing, polishing and serving the guests who had booked accommodation there, and generally doing any job that needed doing. I was paid a pittance by today's standards though was happy enough. I continued to have working holidays at the farmhouse, and later as cupid and fate worked hand in hand I became engaged to the farmer's son. Love will have its way! Five years on and after a brief spell in teaching we were married. As the family then started to arrive, teaching was put on the back burner. My working life again revolved around the tourists who frequented the hamlet, along with my own growing brood of children. Fifty years later I am now a widow. My family are grown and grandchildren are on the scene. I am still here and continue to have an active part working in the tea room, amongst the ever increasing number of visitors. My work and family have been my life. Over the years, as in many businesses, there have been problems: there have been setbacks with loans; overdrafts; weeks when poor weather has resulted in low turnover; long back-breaking hours of work; no mains electricity in the hamlet until 1978 - the list goes on. However I cannot recall anything quite as soul-destroying as the foot and mouth outbreak.

When the epidemic broke I was in Benidorm enjoying a winter break. The only problem I had to consider at this time was would I manage my luggage at the airport as I was travelling alone. I had indulged myself on the holiday and had extra baggage to carry. Whilst away, I had phoned home several times to my daughter. She told me what was happening but the full impact didn't register. It was hard to imagine the whole picture, being so far away and in a relaxed holiday atmosphere. On arrival back home I soon realised how bad the situation and its implications were.

The media was giving full coverage to the crisis with Cumbria seemingly taking the brunt of the virus. For me this was very serious. The holiday euphoria had now receded and was replaced by ever-increasing worry about our livelihood. The business was now one hundred percent closed. There was just no income. The car-park and toilets had been closed, while the road to

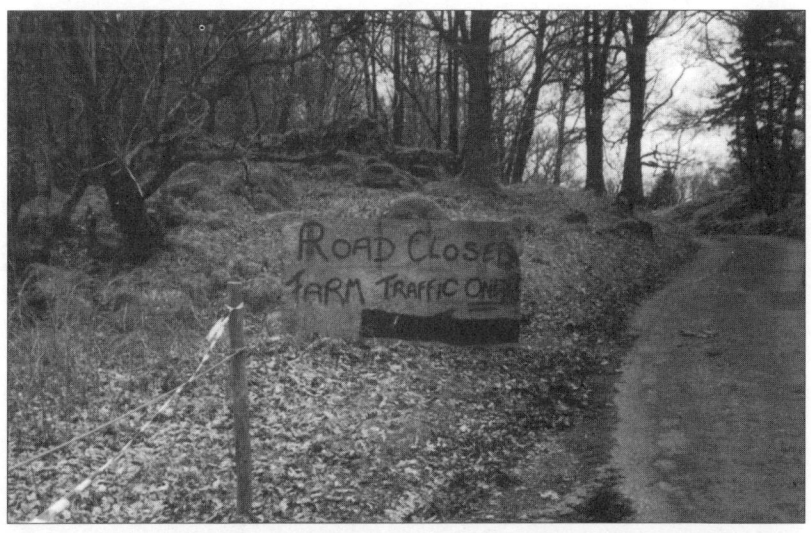

the hamlet displayed signs suggesting that only farm traffic was to proceed. The hamlet was silent. The paths and fells were empty. There wasn't a tourist in sight. The only sounds were the quacking ducks as they foraged for tit-bits in the grass or the birds roosting in the eves of the empty barns. The pot-bellied pig, Thomas, was now confined to a solitary existence in his compound away from his adoring public. Even the spring sunshine and flower beds of healthy daffodils could not dispel the atmosphere of depression that blanketed the hamlet. This eerie silence and air of gloom never lifted. How could such a perfect place exude such a threatening despair? I have recorded this event in photographs. My grandchildren in later years will be able to reminisce about this time and its part in the Watendlath story. Hopefully this episode will never be seen again. The pictures show the deserted road, the empty tea garden and the beautiful scenery bathed in spring sunshine, which at that time no one was able to appreciate.

Day followed day, then week upon week with no change either in the spreading of the virus or the possibility of opening the tea shop. As time went on I was getting more and more depressed and disillusioned. News reports were conflicting, opinions were bandied about, ideas as to how to contain the disease were mulled over yet the virus continued its rampage of destruction through the county. My son and daughter who work with me were feeling the full financial impact of a closed business. I was regularly making phone calls to various individuals and help-lines, and filling in forms and writing letters, as well as attending meetings and going on protest walks. At times these efforts seemed to no avail. I seemed to be getting nowhere. I was getting negative responses. I joined Cumbria Crisis Alliance in Keswick. Members were all business people whose livelihoods had been affected by the foot and mouth and were striving to keep financially afloat. It was good to talk to people with similar problems. We could support each other. Activities within the group were organised to boost morale. For most people, myself included, that was at an all-time low. The Alliance was a real strength.

I felt many emotions during the early weeks. Anger, bitterness, resentment and real aggression. On reflection I attribute this to the fact that I was fighting for my business. I became completely focussed on the crisis. I read every available news report and watched every television bulletin and debate. The words *contiguous, hefted flocks, burning pyres, pits, culled* and *compensation* were part of my everyday vocabulary. I had only one topic of conversation. When in the car I was constantly on the lookout for wagons carrying livestock and driven by men in white coats. These visible pictures were living proof of the catastrophe that was engulfing our lives.

Physically I felt utterly drained and exhausted. I had neither motivation nor money to go anywhere or do anything. I suffered nights of broken sleep and spent many tearful evenings. The worry of the situation took its toll. By this time I was also eating for comfort. We did have confectionery which was going out of date – a lame excuse considering I had previously been trying to follow a weight programme.

After 81 days of full closure, in which time we sold one Mars Bar to the farmer's grandson, we were allowed to reopen. We were euphoric! Disregarding how low the takings might be, we were just so pleased to be open. The tearoom had a part to play again - money was what was needed, and work was the answer. I heaved a sigh of relief, perhaps we could survive. My personal life has, as in most families, seen good times and bad. I have come through them, though not unscathed. I decided that foot and mouth was not going to wipe me out. Why should my working life, through no fault of my own, finish in this way? Being realistic and with all the will in the world, the future of the business is still uncertain. We'll see. I live in hope. Surely, to quote the Labour anthem, 'Things can only get better'. Up to now this year has certainly been my *annus horribilis*.

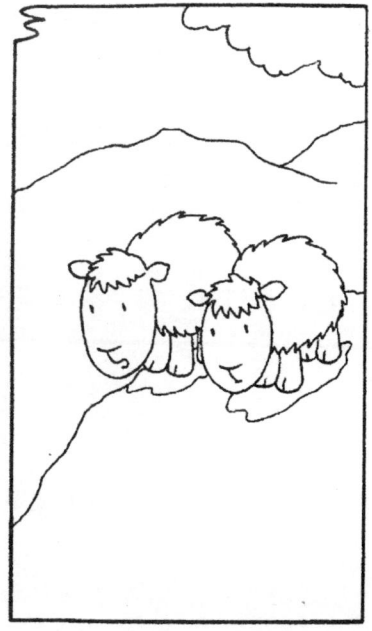

"There aren't as many humans about this Easter .....
Do you think there's something wrong with them?"

Sir Chris Bonington

Sir Chris Bonington, mountaineer, writer and photographer lives in the North Cumbrian fells. He launched the Cumbria Community Recovery Fund Appeal which will receive all profits from the sales of this book.

A climber's experience of the foot and mouth disease crisis

I was driving back from Manchester Airport at the end of March after a climbing trip in the Atlas Mountains of Morocco. I always have a sense of huge elation as I drive through the Howgill Gap. For me it's the gateway to the Northern Lakes. But this time I had a sense of foreboding of what I was going to find as I got nearer to home. Those forebodings were realised all too soon. It was like driving into a war zone, with the heavy pall of smoke from fires on all sides, the stench of rotting corpses and the empty fields.

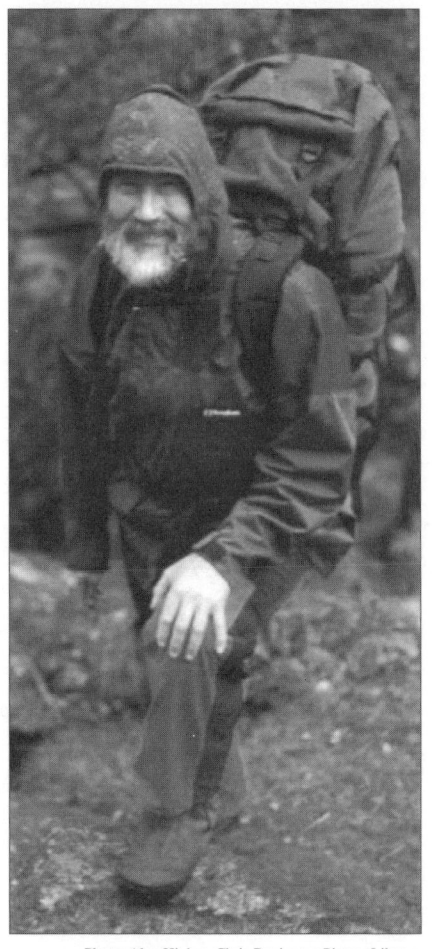

Photo: Alan Hinkes, Chris Bonington Picture Library

It was the height of the crisis in North Cumbria, before Brigadier Birtwistle took charge and when at last there seemed some sense of direction in the fight to contain this dreadful disease. We live on the fell above Caldbeck at the end of winding lane in a little cluster of houses, which were once farms and now the homes of people like ourselves. There is just one exception – a small working farm that nestles closest to the fell.

The factor I most value in where we live is its access to the open fell – the fact that we can wander straight out onto these gentle lovely hills, usually with dog or dogs. I think I must have climbed High Pike a thousand times in the last twenty five years and I never tire of the views across the Eden Valley to the east and the Solway Firth to the north-west. We haven't been on those fells for six months and I miss them grievously, but my sense of loss is of little significance compared to the very real heartache, worry and financial suffering of our neighbours whose livelihoods are affected by the outbreak.

I shall always remember the fight our neighbour has waged to save his little herd of pedigree cattle, his frustration at the lack of information and conflicting directives from MAFF, the struggle of friends in the village involved in the tourist industry with sales down, no one coming to stay. My own frustration seems of little relevance compared to this.

Returning to the Central Lakes once they were opened up at the end of July, what was noticeable was how lush the grass seemed and how many wild flowers there were because of course there were less sheep around. I do hope we learn something from the tragedy of foot and mouth – just how interrelated tourism and farming are. How important farming is to the fabric of the Lake District, but also the need for changes in the way that it is supported so that hill farmers can make a decent living as stewards of the land, with less sheep on the fell, but being able to sell them for a good price as produce of Cumbria.

Most of all I am looking forward to walking up High Pike for the first time in months to the sound of skylarks and stonechats and to sit on the slate seat on the summit and gaze out at that magnificent view of this very special corner of England.

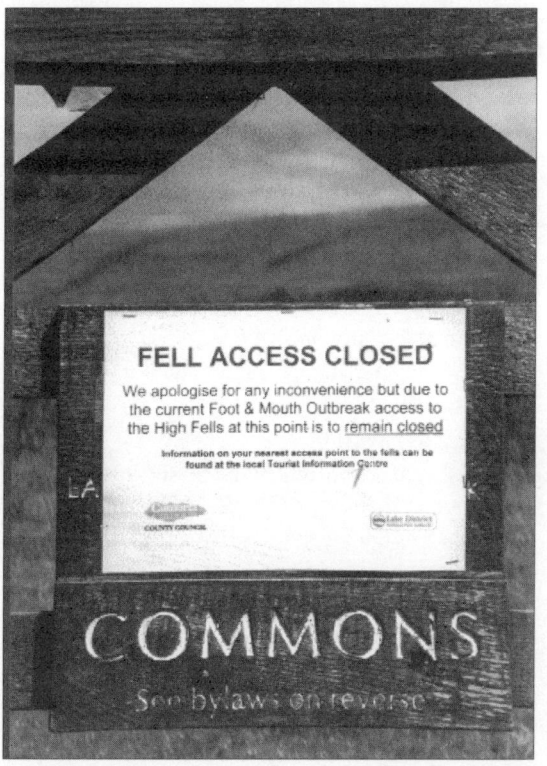

Margaret Buckle

Margaret Buckle has spent her whole life farming in and around Barras, near Kirkby Stephen. When foot and mouth hit Cumbria it became apparent that March 2001 would be like no other. This is her diary.

Sunday 25th February 2001 – Buckles Farm
Movement of animals in Cumbria has stopped because of foot and mouth disease. We all are living in fear as disinfectant mats are put down at farm entrances.

Thursday 1st March
Our away wintered sheep are not allowed to be brought back onto the farm. What about the lambing ewes due towards the end of the month? Those at Winton we have to lamb ourselves. David is not going anywhere near them. John and Jane at Spennymoor are willing to lamb those we have there. Rob and Pat Dickson near Guisborough do not have time to lamb the 280 ewes we have there. What can we do – leave them to fend for themselves? I don't think so – what about me going? I asked husband Derrick and sons Wilf and Kevin. Nothing was said. A woman of almost 64 years old. Should I be doing this? But I asked my almost 62 year old retired sister if she would be willing to come with me and she agreed.

Wednesday 21st March
It is actually happening, made lists of what we need and the caravan of Peter's arrived.

Thursday 22nd March
Alice and I baking in the morning, enough to keep us as long as our stay may be, with a little for Derrick left at home. Vacuumed caravan out and washed it. Only one more night in my own bed for a while. Do I want to do it? Yes, we have to go and help those ewes; everyone else is needed at home. What a mess this foot and mouth has put upon us.

Friday 23rd March
Alice and I had our hair cut and blown-dry at 8.30 a.m. Is that really important? Packed all into trailer and caravan. Gave the house a final clean up. Going to miss my grandchildren and it includes Rachel's and Matthew's birthdays. Taking my Mother's Day cards and fruit, plants and cakes with us. Johnny fixing lights etc. for us. Phone calls and people wishing us well. Peter up to see how we are doing. Says not to worry about anyone bothering us as no one will want us two old b…..'s! Heard Janet Wood on the radio giving her views about it all, she ended by

saying it brings a lump to your throat and a tear to your eyes and I say much more. When will we be home?

Saturday 24th March

Alice here by 10 a.m. for final packing. Left at 11.30 a.m. – Alice's Terrano and trailer, Land Rover and caravan. Derrick and Kevin and Johnny setting us up. Arrived at 12.45. Rob and Pat came to welcome us. Set caravan up and tarpaulin across to trailer. Had sandwiches and coffee. Derrick and Johnny went to put electric sheep fence up so that we can move sheep out as they lamb. Kevin and us walked around field to look at ewes. They are fit but ground is wet. Put three lambs into other field. 11 lambs in lambing field. Injected ewe for staggers. D, J and K had a coffee then went home at 4.15 p.m. It was rather sad to see them go. Looked around sheep at 5.45 p.m. One lamb dead on muck heap. Prepared supper then looked around again. Alice baited fox with dead lamb. 7 p.m. sausage, egg, tomato for supper. 7.30 p.m. Herald to read.

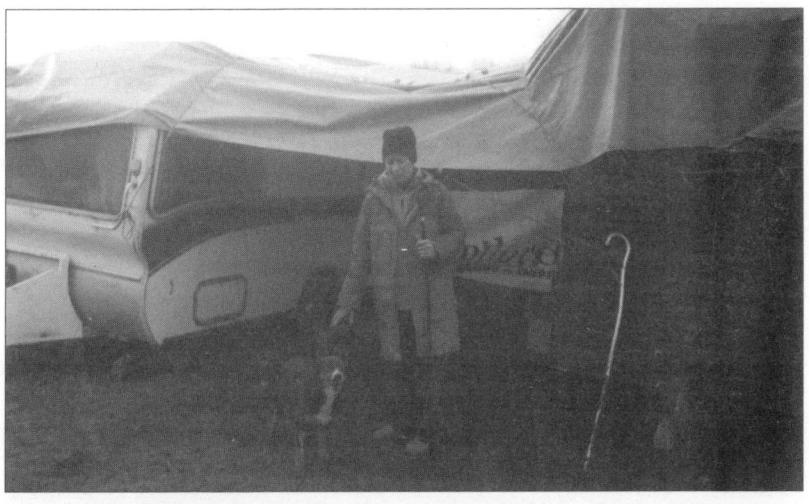

Alice with Spot the sheepdog outside their new makeshift home

Sunday 25th March

Up at daybreak, slept well and warm. Twins born overnight, put them into lamb hospital and 1 single lamb born too. Breakfast at 8.15 a.m. - orange juice and 2 slices toast and marmalade. Car with 4 lads came down lane but went away. Looked sheep around again, put morning's single into other field. Rob and Pat down to feed, they are coming back to fence off bridge so that we can get the sheep into other field easier. Brought one ewe that had single in. It had another not so good. Died later. Roast beef, veg and gravy with blackcurrant pie to follow. Cup coffee and bun at 3.15. Cold and damp. Brought 3 ewes and lambs into pens out of little field marked, tailed and castrated. Then took 3 ewes off lambing field and did same. Did same of 2 in shed ready for Rob to trailer into field tomorrow morning. Alice took dead lamb and baited another fox snare. Her skills are many. She also tailed the gimmer lambs for me while I held them. Not a bad Mother's Day for us, 4 cards, plant, fruit and cakes. What more do we want? Sausage and beans for supper. Not a minute to spare. Don't know what it will be like when they are lambing fast. Last time around, No.1 in little field, ewe wandering off. Came back for bottle of milk and injection penicillin. Would not suck. Put coat on it. Back in at 8.10 p.m., dark. Found alarm clock. The glasses are on the table. Only for medicinal purposes, of course!

Monday 26th March

Up at 6.20 a.m. Sunny, slight frost. No lambs. No.1 dead. We wash with water from our hot water bottles. Rob and Pat came and took our water can to fill. They can't do enough. 7 lambs marked etc. and into grass, only one old lamb left to get out. Spot, the old sheepdog we brought with us is doing well but she is so unhappy. Got last old lamb marked and out. Gelded 3 Swaledales - hope they would not make tups. Put twins and a single into shed. Richard put some big bales into lamb field for shelter. Can see the farmstead from our caravan and busy traffic on A171. Drier day but it is rather cold. Pat pointed out Captain Cook's monument and Roseberry Topping nearby. Homemade meat and vegetable pie for supper. Dark at 8 p.m. tonight.

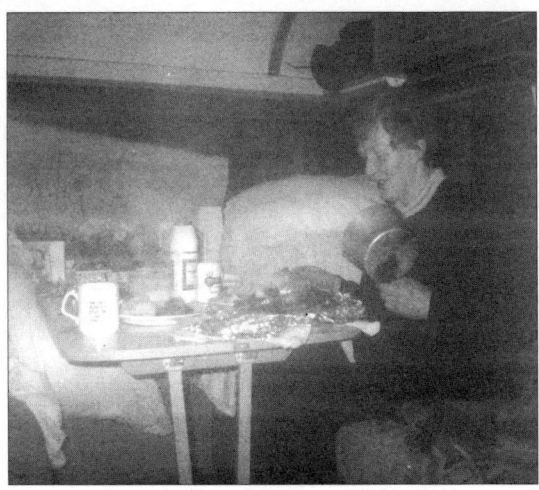

Supper time

Had a 15-minute walk in wood and walked big field fence down wood side filling in holes with bits of wood and old posts. Derrick on phone 9 p.m. seems a little worried about it all. Thinks it is bad that we are having to do this.

Tuesday 27th March
Out at 6.30 a.m. Spot had a bad night dreaming and uneasy. She woke me up as she put her nose on my face then went across to Alice and cried. Wish I had brought Derrick's coat for her to lie on. Single lamb and dead twins first thing. Cold and dry. Ewe of single down with staggers in hospital, fed lamb the bottle. Ewe recovered. Pat took our washing. Caked ewes and lambs, good to see the lambs chasing each other while the ewes feed. A duck and drake have adopted us. Walked down into the wood, dug a hole near a swamp and buried from the chemical toilet. What we have to do! Roast beef and tomato sandwiches for lunch. Afternoon cup coffee after coming in from being around sheep, putting one out into little field. Carried a big bale of old haylage and spread it out on approach to pen gate as it is so muddy. Knocked a post and stapled wire to it at a weak spot in big field. Lamber down with staggers. Up 2 hours later. Roast lamb, potatoes and carrots for supper, crackers and cheese. Strong wind and lashing rain. I do hope we can save these sheep and enjoy our own lamb sometime in the future. Seem to be miles from home and our families. Going out again at 7 p.m. to push lambs into shelter and last look around lambers.

Wednesday 28th March
Wind and rain stopped. First thing 2 with staggers, brought new twins into hospital. At dark last night Pat and Rob brought our clean towels back. What a wonderful couple. This caravan of Peter's is such a luxury. Another wonderful person. My adopted son. Looked around lambs and field. Fox has gone with dead lamb and lamb No. 12. Here we are trying to save these sheep for the fox to eat. I think all those against fox-hunting do not understand in the least. Feeling for those at home as our 100 plus gimmer hoggs at Abbeytown go for cull in the 2 mile radius. Wax jacket over fence drying, also my jumper. Bright at the moment. Topped up with milk, twins in hospital. Lamb and tomato sandwiches for lunch. My teeth feel fresh, soaked them in Steredent last night. Want for nothing here. Our set up looks like a gypsy camp. As a matter of interest and for the record a toilet roll has lasted 4 days!

Thursday 29th March
Three new lambs first thing. Fine and milder. I will never listen again to

anyone who says everyone is so selfish these days and only think of themselves – not these people at Upsall Grange. Ian the farm worker brought us lots of hurdles before lunch. Spent the afternoon making pens ready in case we have lots to bring in. 11 pens made. Opened our first loaf of vacuum-packed bread. Very tasty with our own mustard and pork sausage. Castaways? No, we think casted away. Sausage and onion omelets for tea followed by peaches and custard. Tasty. Mild this evening but some nasty showers.

Friday 30th March

8 lambs first thing. Triplets. Brought them in, and twins. Bottled them. Rob and Pat gave us permission to go into Guisborough, so we went for gas and bread, disinfecting our feet and wheels on leaving the field and on returning. Got a few strange looks, maybe they thought we were Romany folk. The shopkeepers were very kind. Treat ourselves to a huge cheese bread and circle of iced buns, which we had for lunch. A walk down the wood with my spade and slop bucket. 17 lambs mid afternoon. Sunny. Charging the battery up off Alice's motor for lights in our caravan. Our towels have dried out, pegged onto the rope that is fastening the tarpaulin. I think we have someone looking over us all the time. This morning Pat was telling us someone she knows had forecast what will happen on their farm. Alice looked down and there on the ground was a small wooden cross. She picked it up and hung it on our hospital shed. It gave us hope. We saw daffodils bursting into flower on our way to Guisborough. Spring is around. Ended up with 18 lambs today. Pasta, tomatoes and tuna for supper followed by apple pasty and custard.

Saturday 31st March

Been here 7 full days. 5 lambs first thing then 3 more later. Keeping triplets in for another day, although topping up with bottle. After coffee had to lamb one coming backwards. Roseberry had lambed also. You know, this foot and mouth has put extra pressure on Rob and Pat. They have had to patch up fences for our sheep that should have been home with us at Buckles Farm on 1st March. 3 fields have been put aside for the sheep whereas they would normally have been cut 3 or 4 times. Hope and pray that the gimmers we are helping to face this world will be future breeding stock. 11 lambs this afternoon. We both just had to go to the hairdressers. It's only a few strides from our base. In fact, on the field edge, washing from one bucket, rinsing from another. Used water left in buckets to wash a few clothes which are now drying on the fence with towels. The ewe I lambed coming backwards had another and we brought them into hospital. Fox went with lamb No. 18. To recognise these sheep, when we can finally take them home, we are spray marking the ewes and lambs with green behind their heads. When we have a wagon load we will change colour.

Sunday 1st April
3 pair twins and 4 singles first thing and it is fine. Listened to gospel choruses for half hour at 6 a.m. on BBC Radio Cleveland while we had a cup of coffee. It lifted us for a start to the day. April fool? There are no fools down here. Even the ewes in hospital have 4 star treatment: haylage, sweet meadow hay, ewe rolls and mixture, water and a roof over their heads. What a menu! Injected 3 with Maxacal. One had got in a deep-water gutter and she is weak. Pat is taking our weekly washing to do. A welcome sight seeing the Land Rover at the end of the lane with Kevin, my son, spraying it with disinfectant. Pleased to see Derrick after 8 days and Jack. I think they thought we looked well and were doing a good job. They had lunch and tea with us and looked around the sheep and helped us to drive those that had lambed onto big field. Departed at around 4.30 p.m. 19 lambs today.

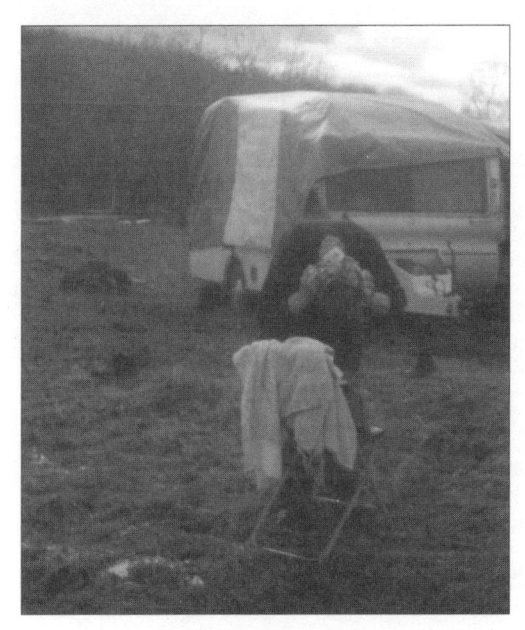

Hair-washing alfresco.

Monday 2nd April
Fine morning, only 2 lambs. Spot settled down well after seeing Derrick yesterday. Shall be forever grateful to Peter for his caravan. It is a lot more comfortable than if the trailer had been our living quarters. Our own pork chops for lunch followed by homemade apple pie and custard. This morning Alice and I made easier access over a fence into big field by removing the barbed wire and putting a hurdle there for us to climb over. Learnt the sizes of our fields. Lambing field 15 acres. Little field $4^1/_2$ acres. Big field 11 acres. A fair walk around many times each day. Put

LIST OF WHAT IS NEEDED

SELF	DAY TO DAY REQ.	SHEEP
Trousers	Bin bags	Disinfectant
Jumpers	Matches	Brush
Shirts	Gas	8 Hurdles
Pants	Jenny	12 posts
Socks	Petrol	Roll wire fencing
Hat	Torches	Post hammer
Scarf	Candles	Gavelek
Gloves	Tea towels	Spade
Waterproof overalls	Foil	Hammer
Waterproof jacket	Kitchen roll	Pincers
Wellies	Dish cloth	Nails
Trainers	Water container	Staples
Sleeping bag	Bucket	Tarpaulin
Duvet	Washing up liquid	Bag bale string
Pillow	Domestos	2 Shepherds crooks
Sheet	Toilet chemical	Buckets
Hairbrush	Washing liquid	Dog feed
Shampoo	Pans	Dog bowls
Glasses	Kettle	Lamb milk
Magazines	Basins	Lamb bottle
Towels	Plates	Lamb teats
Face cloth	Mugs	Rubber gloves
Soap	Tin opener	Pocket knife
Toothbrush	Cutlery	Lambing diary
Toothpaste	Sherry and glasses	Footrot shears
Steredent	Dustpan and brush	3 syringes
Hot water bottles	Cooking oil	Needles
Biro	Sugar	Stomach pump
Diary	Salt	Terramycin
Plasters	Coffee	Maxacal
Vaseline	Tea bags	Pennicillin
Painkillers	Marmalade	Curved needle & thread
Scissors	Jam	Aerosol marking tins
Alarm clock	Ryvita	Iodine
Lypsil	Marg. Spread	Straw
Toilet rolls	Crackers	Hay
2 garden chairs	Biscuits	Roughtex
Radio	Tinned fruit & veg	
Mobile telephone	Pasta	
	Potatoes	

triplets and twins out of hospital into the little field. One of each had split away at teatime but got them together again. Don't know what their chances are of keeping together. The ewe that had been injected many times and got into the ditch, died. Saw a butterfly this afternoon.

Tuesday 3rd April
7 lambs first thing. Got 11 lambs marked. Fine morning. Going to stop caking ewes with lambs so they don't get split up. Rob down and he said he would put a feeder in and give them hay or silage to chew at if they wanted it. As NFU chairman of his local branch, this morning he is fighting to stop whoever is organising it from bringing welfare slaughtered pigs from Witton le Wear onto a pit-burial on our doorstep at Guisborough, into a non-infected area. Spare lamb in field, so it will become a pet. Can't see what it belongs to. Old ewe died, did not respond to treatment. It was mother of lamb No. 22, so 2 pet lambs. Day for going into the woods with my spade. A job that has to be done. Just thought, poor Rob, 10 days ago was leading a peaceful life with one woman in his life. Tammy, his daughter-in-law, came home to have her baby and Alice and I landed on his farm. 4 women to contend with now! Too many ewes down, and one is not very good tonight. Alice found the remains of a lamb, its front leg in little field. Another one for Mr. Fox. I wish those against fox-hunting could see what the fox is doing to our lambs and the distress it causes the ewe.

Wednesday 4th April
What a morning! We are flooded out. Only twins this morning, which we have put inside. What we would have done without this shed I don't know. It's geared up for paintballing. Rob lets it out for a day at a time to groups. Phone call from Kevin. The Ministry wants to speak to them this morning about the cull of our Abbeytown gimmer hoggs. Had a word with all the kids except Matthew. One of our pet lambs died this morning. Had to lamb one that was stuck, what a big lamb. Its head and tongue were very swollen so we brought it in. Having a rock bun that we baked 2 weeks ago. We vacuum-packed them and they taste as if they were freshly baked. Pat brought our coats and gloves back that she had been drying for us. Alice has various names for sheep connected with someone she knows. There is May, Sheila, Jack and Roseberry.

Thursday 5th April
Fine morning. Marked etc. yesterday's lambs. Fox has been and got lamb No.18. It's the second No. 18 it has taken. Cleaned wet straw out of pens that were flooded yesterday. Ian, Rob's farm worker (a grand lad), said

we only need a horse and then we would be part of the travelling folk. No. 18 lamb's mother has had so much stress fighting the fox off last night she has also died. There was the lamb dead with all its tail bitten off and torn flesh at its neck. Its mother had not allowed the dead lamb to be dragged away by the fox.

Friday 6th April
Marked yesterday's and looked at those that have lambed. They are looking really good and healthy. Pleased with what we have lambed up till now, only wish the ones that are left would get a move on. Went into Guisborough for bread etc. Sent Easter cards home and Wilf a birthday card. Repaired a fence down near shed. Pat and Rob down as always every day. They never show that it is a nuisance us being here and can't do enough for us. I do hope that some way we can show kindness to them. No. 74 has got split up from its mother and twin so brought it in and will try and get it to go back tomorrow.

Saturday 7th April
9 lambs this morning. Brought one lot of twins in. It has been heavy rain last night and they were wet and dirty. Ewe was wild but Spot was there. She has been brilliant for us and has recovered fully from her operation and is not crying and dreaming of Derrick and home anymore. Put 3 sets of twins into hospital. The wind and rain is atrocious, not fit for man or beast. Could be putting on weight even though we are walking the fields often. We start the day at 5.30 a.m. with coffee and biscuit, breakfast is orange juice, 2 slices toast and marmalade, tea. Coffee time, we have coffee and cake. Lunch is a cooked meal, crackers and cheese, tea. At tea time it's coffee and cake. And for supper, sandwiches, custard and fruit. Alice saw a fox in next field this morning.

Sunday 8th April
Our tup we shared with Gill Gate at Askrigg had to be culled. Raining when we went to bed last night, everything white with frost this morning. Very bright now and sunny. Church bells greeted us from the distance at 8 a.m. in one direction then at 9 a.m. in another. 9 lambs this morning, including Sheila's twins as slim as her. Rob and Pat had been to church this morning and said a prayer for us. Hair-washes this afternoon again outside our caravan. Towels drying on the fence. Put my duvet and sheet out to air-fresh. Up to today, we have lost 4 ewes (3 staggers, 1 fox stress). A lamb born first time round at 6 a.m. had been killed by a fox at 9.15 a.m.; its hind legs were left. Yorkshire pudding today for dinner.

Monday 9th April

Fine morning. Got yesterday's lambs marked and out. Doctored 3 of the ewes' feet. The foot and mouth is getting nearer at home and Rachel, my daughter-in-law, told us that they would have to be monitored. Alice has her mobile phone and it is good to be in contact with home. Spoke to the kids yesterday, they are missing us and we are missing them. Wilf's birthday today. Our toast today is from a loaf of bread that we vacuum-packed 3 weeks ago at home. Tastes fine, although a little squashed. 8 lambs this morning. Pat has washed our bedding today and brought it back down ready for use tonight. She is full of kindness. We also got home-made cake and bread. We were told our Blonde bull that David Cannon had borrowed had to be culled.

Tuesday 10th April

Foggy, damp and cold wind this morning. Up at 5.15 a.m. 6 lambs. Morning for going into the wood with the spade. Around the fields with lambs in, just to check. Rachel on phone saying our animals at home had been examined by the Ministry, because the milk tanker had been on an infected farm. Richard and Rob down to see that we are OK. Spoke to Derrick on the phone.

Wednesday 11th April

Foggy, damp and cold wind. Brought yesterdays single in, ewe had a big teat. 6 lambs this morning. 12.30 a.m. and the fox has bitten the tail off a lamb and bitten its mouth off and left it dead. Just lambed one. It was coming correct but was dead on arrival. Going down hill as far as eating is concerned. From rib of beef down to battered spam as our provisions run down. Rob has brought us some of Henry Brewis's funny stories of sheep to keep our spirits up. Very worried for those back home, they are very much in amongst it all. Feel as if I should be back home just to be there for them. Treated the Suffolk tup to a pedicure, trimmed its feet and cut off all the muck around its backend.

Thursday 12th April

What a start to the day. Home-made bread and lemon curd. First prize to both. Thank you Pat! White with frost this morning. 6 lambs first thing. 3 lots of twins to get out of big field through sheep electric fence, so Spot had to round them up. Brought in 2 lots of twins that were cold.

Friday 13th April - Good Friday

Fine and sunny, no wind this morning. No lambs. Good Friday. Have an arrangement of Palm in the pot with the Mothers' Day primroses to celebrate Easter. Lots of caravans we can see going yesterday and today on A171 towards Whitby. Had our lunch sitting outside. Again, home-made bread and cake from Pat. All out of hospital except April and May, our pets.

Saturday 14th April

2 lambs first thing. Weather fine but a little cold. Down into the wood with the spade this morning. Went into Guisborough for shopping, gas shop was closed. Cream cake treat for tea. One or two are getting out into greener pastures so we have been filling up holes. Their motto is 'don't fence me in'. Can't contact home as Pat took the mobile phone to get charged. Did speak to Derrick later as Rob brought the phone back.

Sunday 15th April - Easter Sunday

Bright sunny morning. Put yesterday's out into little field. One ewe was an awkward beggar. Easter Sunday - wonder what it will bring? I think these ewes are having an Easter break. Feel rather sad and lonely as I usually organise an Easter ramble for my grand-children and the local children. But the family at Upsall Grange has given us a very appropriate Easter card. Well chosen, a picture of a sheep with a flower in its mouth plus a box of Thorntons' chocolates. Pat is also sending our Sunday lunch down. Their kindness to others I know some day will be rewarded. Richard and David brought our lunch as promised and it was some lunch, 4 star class. Wonderful! Thank you Pat! We may be a long way from home but we have not missed out, in fact, we have some of our lunch left that will make a lovely sandwich for supper. Reflecting on the past 3 weeks on what has kept us sane: I think the daily contact by phone to back home, Pat's kindness with home-made bread and cakes, Easter Sunday lunch, Easter card and chocolates and Rob's humour with his photocopied jokes. Alice and I also laugh at each other at some of the stupid things we do. A very happy day, if one can be happy.

Monday 16th April - Easter Monday

Cold North wind, sleet showers. At 8 a.m. as we went to feed the pet lambs, there as brazen as brass, was a fox just 50 yards from our caravan. It slinked slowly away back into the woods. Rob brought a vixen and dog fox that Simon (a lad he knows) had shot last night at midnight in the field with lambs in. Well done Simon! Caravans are starting to move back home after the Easter break. Well, this day and time next week we should be back home. The longest I've been away from home is 2 weeks and by the time we get home from here it will be 4 weeks and 2 days from home. No matter what age you are one never knows what you might come up against in life.

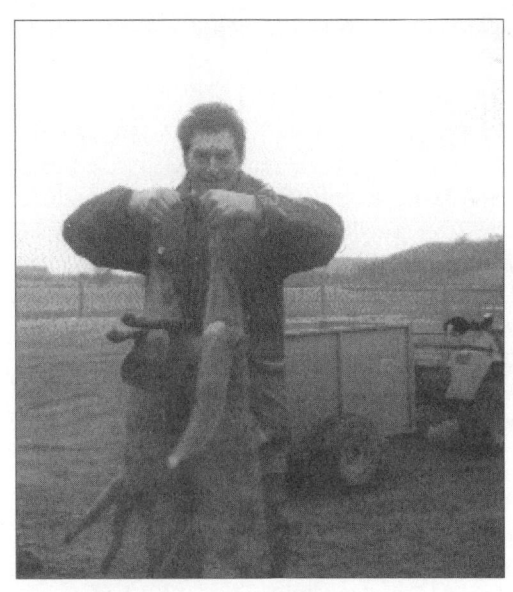

Rob and the foxes

Tuesday 17th April
Fine frosty morning. 2 lambs and 2 ewes lambing first time around. Had to assist one to lamb next time around. Red 83 lamb was sitting around so gave it a penicillin jab and 2 rattle belly capsules. Went into Guisborough for gas after we had our soup and roll. Washed my hair, won't do it again until we get home. 8 p.m. and just got in from last look around. Absolutely pouring down and windy. Auntie Eleanor called us on the phone and said they were all thinking of us. It was sweet of her.

Wednesday 18th April
As we opened our caravan curtains at 5.30 a.m. snow on the ground outside confronted us It is a cold strong wind also. The weather here has been so bad. I have not once been able to walk around the sheep without my overalls or coat. There's lots of wildlife for us to watch; deer, fox, pheasants, ducks, moorhen, partridge, stoats, herons, Canada geese.

Thursday 19th April
Cold dry morning. Nothing doing. Spoke to Derrick, Maria, Stuart and Michelle on phone last night. Everything is bad at home. What is the future for us all? Injected No 83 again with penicillin and it seems a little better. Spent the afternoon taking down our railings in the shed, extending the pet lamb pen and tidying up. Put a couple of wood posts in at corners to tie the electric fence to. Some terrible wintry showers. End of another day nearer to going home.

Friday 20th April
Dry morning but still cold. Found an old lid for the pet lambs to have their Roughtex in. Pat is going to bottle feed them for a week or so until they go out into the field. Sad to leave them but I hope they will come home before long. Treated a few for foot rot. Patched a bit of fence up.

The Suffolk tup is walking better. The first Suffolk lamb appeared. It has been mules until now.

Saturday 21st April

Hard frost and all is white. The sun is shining bright at 9 a.m. and the frost is disappearing. The radio says it is going to cloud up and rain. Thanks, Stuart, for the radio. We have been able to know what has been going on away from us. One from a set of twins died. She has not had a lot of milk. As we are going home on Monday I decided not to bring it in to feed. It was kinder to let it die. There'll be no one here to feed it and I could not have taken it back home with me. Knocked a few staples in at a weak spot in the fence. The two pet lambs got their names written along one side of their body – April and May and a stroke right along their other side. This was with bright orange spray. In afternoon went into the wood and dug a big hole, only one more time to do this job. Alice has been willing to do any job this past four weeks except this one. Lovely quiet night.

Sunday 22nd April

Dry morning. Simon called 8.30 p.m. last night with the fox's brush; he had got another one. Saved another lamb by being here. The lamb was coming backwards and was stuck. Pat gave us permission to take some rare plant that is growing in a swamp in the wood; we will try to grow it at home. Have packed a few things away into Alice's motor ready for off

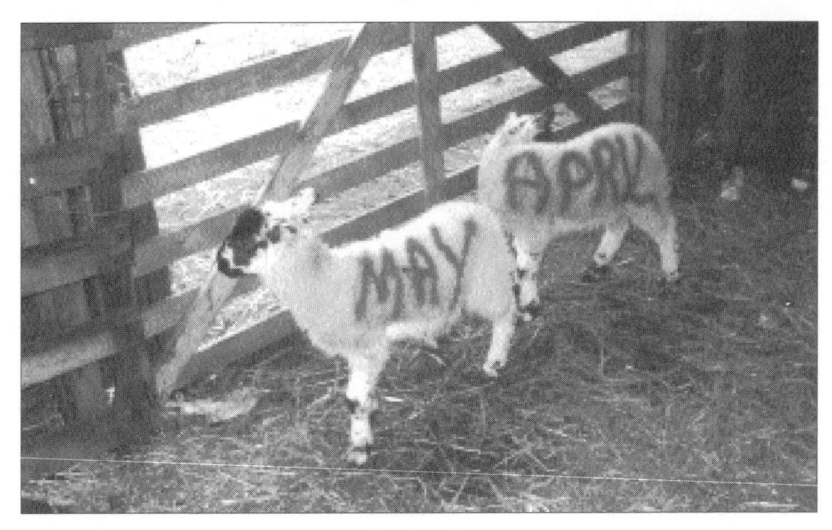

Pet lambs

tomorrow. Will have to leave the trailer at Upsall Grange Farm because no one can come for it because of the situation back home. It is too risky when the disease is so near. Moved sheep from one field to the other while Richard spread fertilizer on all three fields. It will give us chance to see that all are mothered up in the morning. Saw Simon on his way into the wood seeking foxes.

Monday 23rd April

Fine morning. Simon into the wood looking for foxes at 5.30 a.m. Took tarpaulin off without any difficulty. Put it in trailer to come home later. Rob is taking the trailer into his farmyard as he says if it was left down this lane it would be stolen in a short time. Goodbye to our pet lambs April and May. All packed up. Last look around all sheep, put last 3 lambs out into other field after rubber ringing etc. Sad to leave them after being in our care for 4 weeks. Hitched onto the caravan. Said thank you and goodbye to Pat and Rob and set off home at 3 p.m. Warm welcome from Wilf, Maria and kids at Bleathgill road end. Home to balloons and a lovely tea. Spot was happy to see Derrick, as was I. Rachel told us friends and relatives asking how we were getting on had phoned her. How kind people are. Little Tom could not walk when we left but he is going like a good one now. There were only three items we had missed off our list and could have done with – pepper, air freshener and worm dosing as 3 or 4 ewes were skittered out, but gave them a jab of penicillin. Don't know if that will help at all.

Derrick thinks we did well with the number of lambs we lost. 4 dead when born, 4 killed by foxes and 4 various other reasons.

NO ENTRY: Animal Disease Control Precautions

Lord Inglewood MEP

As a farmer, landlord and landowner Lord Inglewood, who represents Cumbria and the North West in the European Parliament, was hit by the full force of the foot and mouth outbreak. Five of his farms were infected by the disease.

I didn't think much about foot and mouth. There had been a bit when I was a child of course, but I didn't really remember it, and there were odd outbreaks in Europe in places like Greece. And then suddenly it was in Essex, and they said it came from that derelict looking farm I used to see at Heddon on the way to Newcastle Airport.

Next it was jumping to Longtown, to Sockbridge, and to Newton Rigg. It was on our doorstep. From then on it was all in the hands of the gods. We all knew it in our hearts. I expect I must have felt a bit like my father on the perimeter at Dunkirk in 1940.

It was a telephone call just after 9 a.m. on a Sunday morning 'I'm afraid we've got it at Home Farm' said Andy. We had. MAFF dithered. I thought of the cows the other side of the trees and John and his family and Simon shut in, and the killing and the burning. Two weeks later Whitrigg Farm went, and then New Rent, the young stock - that was the worst, and Eric and his family had been living in effective isolation for weeks.

I was the boss and I couldn't see or do anything, excluded by MAFF, but at least able to speak in Westminster and Brussels. It helped being on the political front line even though I don't believe either the Authorities or the rest of the country grasped what was happening.

My exposure to the killing fields was down the telephone, the mobile taking me into the carnage. The worst was the joyful crying of the newborn lambs in the lambing shed, the best lambing we have had - knowing that at the same time they were being slaughtered at the other end. I couldn't do a blind thing for real, but I hope it helped talking and listening.

And then a few weeks later it happened again at Wythop, our Hill Farm. The ghastly ritual of destruction once more, but at least by then the burning had stopped.

Why me? Why us? Who knows? God moves in a mysterious way. But the family are all right, so are all those working on the farm. I am not bankrupt. It could have been much worse: it would have been in Kosovo or Bangladesh, or here in the Middle Ages. Self-pity is useless, after all most people in Britain couldn't care less – they have their own immediate and pressing problems.

Get on with it. Other people deal with adversity. Farming is going to change anyway and so it should. Whatever it is, do it better and differently next time. It's taken ospreys 150 years to come back to the Lake District, I can't wait that long, and as for the rest of them ....(the editor told me the rest was unprintable).

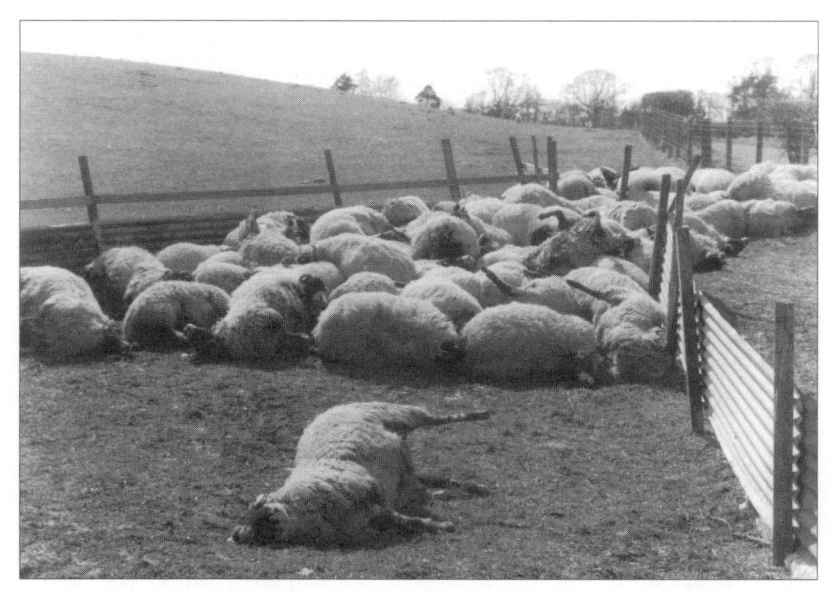

Photo: Nick Green

NO ENTRY: Animal Disease Control Precautions

Gordon L. Routledge

Gordon Routledge was born in Longtown and has lived and worked there all his life. He is also a local historian and writer.

Longtown - the last town in England - as it has been called, in old times nestled on the edge of the Debatable Lands and suffered greatly at the hands of the advancing armies, both English and Scottish, as the Wars of Independence raged on for several centuries. Our small community which sprung up beside the ford on the River Esk has experienced a great deal through the ages including hardship and strife but today its quiet appearance belies its troubled past. Many have settled here through the years, English and Scots, travelling gypsies and Irish who came to work in the now defunct cotton industry, then, more recently, the Dutch who came to work the Solway Moss and the Polish who settled here after the Second World War.

In 1306 a grant was made to hold the first market in the Manor of Arthuret. Longtown was then developed by the Graham family of Netherby and became a thriving market town. Today it is a special community with a life and character of its own. The Longtown market has continued more or less ever since until the recent foot and mouth epidemic which tore the heart out of the community and brought the farming industry to its knees.

I can give an insight into the way things have been in Longtown during the past six months or so from three different angles.

The first one is through my position within the Defence Munitions Depot, Longtown, where Smalmstown Farm, just north of Longtown, and the depot site were the first places in Cumbria to be declared infected areas. One of those strange and inexplicable coincidences is that on 24th of March 1999 in my capacity as Director of Operations D.M. Longtown, I, along with the Commandant Lt. Col. Davison, escorted Brigadier Alex Birtwistle, then of 42 Command Brig. Preston, around the Smalmstown Depot site on a routine visit. This was the only time I ever met the Brigadier, and how strange it seems that he should visit Smalmstown and, by some peculiar quirk of fate, he would be the man that the army would appoint to help stop the spread of the disease two years later, and who would become a household name for the excellent work he did for our region. Smalmstown, meanwhile, became synonymous with foot and mouth disease and was the first farm in Cumbria to have all of its livestock killed. I will never forget seeing all of the animals rounded up on the Friday night and thinking that by Saturday they would all be gone, which indeed they were. The people of Longtown witnessed one gory spectacle after another as pyres burned day and night for weeks on end and the killing went on and on. We were greatly distressed by these events and one night after work I went up to Arthuret Church and stood and looked across the Valley of the Esk. All I could see was smoke rising in every direction throughout the parishes of Arthuret and Kirkandrews and on across the border to Scotland. The area resembled a disaster zone and I realised that I

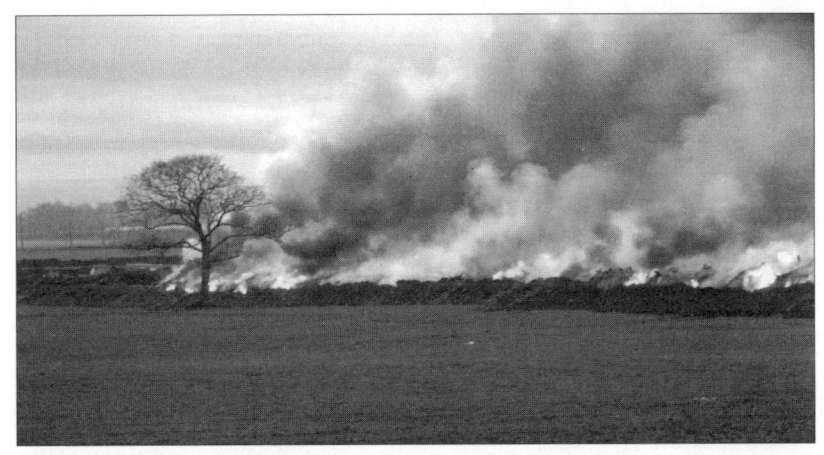

Photo: News & Star

was standing at roughly the same place where Sir Thomas Wharton, the deputy Warden of the English West March, had stood prior to the Battle of Solway Moss in 1542 as he watched the advancing Scottish army burning the Grahams out of the Debatable Lands. I am sure that the scene he witnessed was very similar to that which I was looking out over and that nothing remotely like it had been witnessed since that time.

My second insight into the foot and mouth crisis was in my capacity as an Arthuret Parish Councillor. I attended many meetings about foot and mouth including the never to be forgotten Public Meeting in the Longtown Community Centre on April 11th when the people spoke out with one voice against the burning at Hallburn. A 'super-pyre' had been constructed on the old airfield and the plan was that it should burn 24 hours a day throughout the summer to get rid of the backlog of dead animals. Longtown man, James Bell, posed his thirteen questions to the meeting, the last of which was: 'Is there anything that can be said that will stop the burning at Hallburn?' The following day a decision was taken and the burning ceased. The people, for once, had made a difference.

I also had the opportunity to meet the Environmental Minister, Michael Meacher. We put various questions and concerns to him. I remember mine was on air quality monitoring and the long term effect of burning on the local community. I will always remember Donald Jefferson, our County Councillor, saying that the ministers should come up from London, stand on the Esk Bridge and get the smell of that stuff into their noses then they would know how things were at Longtown. In fact Longtown, whose only claim to fame in recent times, was as the epicentre of the 1979 earthquake, was now the main focus for the world press, through no fault of its own and for all the wrong reasons. It became a regular feature to see camera crews setting up their equipment in the streets of the town or opposite the auction market.

My third perspective on foot and mouth was as a local resident living in Esk Street, Longtown where we experienced the smoke from the pyres and the unbearable stench of burning carcasses day and night. From the rear window of our house the flames from the How End pyre could be seen rising and glowing in the evening sky. In fact we endured that stench all day at work and again in the evenings on returning home and no matter what you did it managed to penetrate any barrier. Double-glazing couldn't keep it out and nobody had their windows open for about six weeks. I remember one local man telling a newspaper how he stuck Selotape over his keyhole in an effort to keep it out. Of course these discomforts were nothing compared to the suffering of the farming community and we shared their sorrow day after day as more and more outbreaks were reported through the media.

Local hardware store owner John Graham, a well known figure in the town, offered to put up Tony Blair and invited him to have a holiday in Longtown. 'He would be welcome to come and stop with me and I think the break would do him good.' John agreed that he would show him round the area and the highlight of the visit would be a Saturday night out in the Robin Hood at Smithfield where he would learn more speaking to the regulars than he would studying at Oxford and Cambridge. They would even buy him a few gin and tonics. Now that would really be something!

The new millennium, which had promised so much, brought with it such devastation. The Rev. John Smith of our local church at Arthuret summed things up most poignantly in a television broadcast where he said that 'Our whole community is hurting.' To me that says it all - but we are a tough community and we will bounce back. In time the economy will recover, the terrible sights and sounds may fade in the memory to an extent, but will never be erased from the minds of those people who lived through it. This was Longtown in the year 2001. It was the year of empty and silent fields and of broken hearts, the year that spring passed us by.

David Maclean

David Maclean is the MP for Penrith and the Border. By mid August when this book was compiled 678 farms in his constituency had become infected premises. That equalled more than a quarter of all cases, almost 550 more than in any other MP's constituency. This is an extract from his diary written near the beginning of the outbreak.

Sunday 18th March, 10 a.m.
A clean, crisp cold but sunny morning in Cumbria with just a few snowflakes. From my desk I look out to the Cumbrian fells and

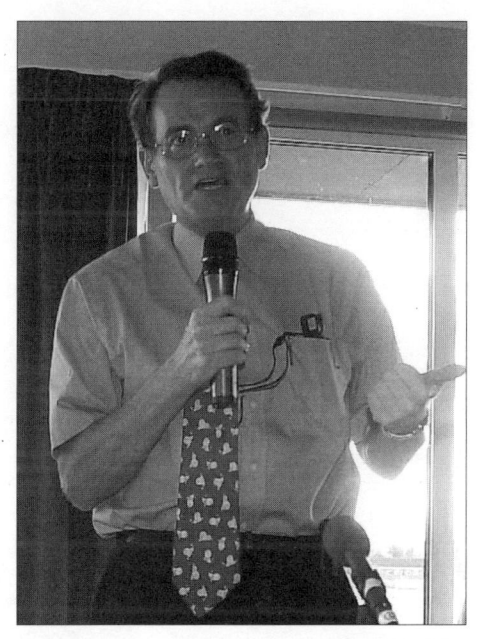

Photo: News & Star

Stobarts Mill in the distance. In my garden two increasingly fat red squirrels have emptied their feed hopper and are chasing each other round the tree and those are the only animals visible in the whole landscape. No sign of any of the thousands of sheep which should cover the rolling hills between my fence and Stobarts Mill. They have not been killed yet just gathered into every barn, clutched tightly into the centre of the farm in a desperate attempt to dodge the virus. I should have been in London today, at the front of the Freedom and Livelihood March. Instead it will be another day telephoning constituents and friends who have not moved outside their door for three weeks and whose livelihood has gone or is about to.

I think of some of the events of the last two weeks and they are all a blur. I look at the fax I sent to some key farming leaders in the constituency a day after the first case was confirmed in Cumbria. I thought it was an overreaction at the time but I have a morbid dread of foot and mouth from my experiences as a boy on a farm in the 60s. It began, 'Gentlemen, I fear we must prepare for the worst. Here are all my contact numbers where you can get me night and day...'

I look at the letters and faxes I sent out, calling for the Army to be called in, for on farm burial, for more vets from around the world. Why is no one listening? I've been there. I've got the MAFF tee shirt. I've been through salmonella, lead poisoning in the West Country, BSE and countless other crises. The Government appointed me to the Board of the Royal College of Veterinary Surgeons, so when I call for all the students from the six University Schools to come out to help, that idea is based on knowledge of the facts.

I look at the 10 Point Plan I sent to the Minister on the 13th. Nothing has happened. I must follow it up if there is to be any hope of saving most of our livestock herds. My secretary has handed me the list of telephone calls and demands for help. The new 'hotline' I have installed records a maximum of 50 calls. It needs to be emptied five times a day at the moment. After the Minister's announcement about the 3 kilometre cull all my lines and faxes have reached melting point. Now I must write again to the Minister and Michael Meacher too, whom I rate.

Still Sunday 18th March but now 10 p.m. What a day! One part of MAFF which has been giving superb service is the Parliamentary Clerk, Christine, who is emailing every MP with the names of farmers hit and the number of cattle and sheep. More have come in today and there is an alarming increase in cattle herds which have no connection with each other. Is it airborne or is it crows and seagulls spreading it? This terrible uncertainty is burning me up, so what is it doing to farmers watching it advance?

One case is three miles from my home. I phone my neighbour Matt who has the champion beef Limousin herd in the County. His voice is a bit flatter than last week and I tell him to hang in there. He, like everyone else, has a million questions I can't answer. BT will make a fortune out of this epidemic. Everyone I try to phone is engaged; farmers are desperate for information; they cannot get out and are constantly phoning everyone they know in a sort of spontaneous helpline system.

I phone my constituency Chairman, not to discuss politics but just to commiserate. His whole herd was due to be slaughtered today. We had already cancelled our AGM because he and others could not move.

I phoned Les Armstrong earlier. He was on the list of farming leaders I sent that first fax to saying that I feared the worst. He phoned me last Saturday. It was a short call, 'It's got me David. I was expecting it.' 'I'm sorry Les', I said. 'So long as it's done quickly', he said. 'I know they've got to go, so let's get it over with and it might stop my neighbours getting it.' 'If there's anything I can do? 'I say, knowing that there isn't. But tonight, a week later I tell him he was statesmanlike on ITV being interviewed from the other side of the barbed wire fence. I also tell him we need him out of quarantine as soon as possible. The County needs farming leadership and it will be good for Les to resume his role as Chairman of the NFU livestock committee as soon as possible.

I've faxed an urgent letter through to Nick Brown asking him to appoint a Supremo to take charge of the deteriorating situation in Cumbria. I also checked with my old army mates to see if it was workable and then faxed in a plan to separate the logistical task of killing, burying and burning from the veterinary job of diagnosis and control. There are still reports of qualified vets spending their time dragging dead sheep around. We must have the Army now.

I prepare a note for Jim Scudamore whom I will meet at 9 o'clock tomorrow in Carlisle. I contacted him last Friday begging him to send a Deputy Chief Veterinary Officer to Cumbria to explain to the local vets why a cull was necessary. Jim phoned me on Friday to say he was coming personally. I admire that.

I've done all the outstanding 'emotional' calls. I must give priority during the day to getting through to offices and writing, faxing and emailing. I have learned the hard way to do all the business calls and faxes during the day and the emotional ones at night. Last Thursday, I left my little Commons office at 1.00 in the morning absolutely drained. What do you say to men, big men with hands like shovels and hearts like an ox who are broken down on the phone? They say, 'Eeh! I canna talk to you any more lad. Can you speak to the wife?' Thank God for the quality of Cumbrian wives. I know that they are holding together so many despairing fathers and sons just now.

Why do they all call me lad? I'm 47 and right now I feel 97.

I must phone Alistair Wannop tomorrow. He is another brilliant young farmer and on my contact list. I need his input on where we go from here.

Monday 19th March. 11 p.m. It's getting worse. The emails keep coming in from Christine at MAFF and more farmers I know have gone down. The knock on to other businesses is astonishing. Jobs are being lost left, right and centre in businesses I did not know exist. The army are coming, I'm told. I wish it was General Havelock and his 5,000 Highlanders to break the Siege of Lucknow but it is only 70 soldiers from the Prince of Wales Own. Too little, too late.

A hundred other things happened today. Each one was important at the time but was, somehow irrelevant two hours later when it was overtaken by even worse news. I have not put down a single Parliamentary Question on this since it is moving so fast that a PQ would need to be answered within two hours or it is out of date.

I had to go down to the Smoking Room and get a large Rusty Nail (half Drambuie, half Malt) to take back to my room before I could continue with the night calls.

I did phone Alistair Wannop today. Not to seek advice though. The email from Christine came through at 7.29 p.m. telling me he was hit. 700 prime dairy cattle. Julie answered the phone and I just couldn't speak. Alistair was out looking at his cattle as I expected.

The cull will not happen, at least not as planned. So many herds are now being hit that they cannot keep up with killing infected animals.

I try to order more telephone lines from BT for my constituency office. BT says it will take ten days. I say it is foot and mouth and I must have them tomorrow. The girl says that I must phone someone in MAFF in Chester and he will authorise priority installation. I ring. He is very helpful. They will be installed tomorrow. Another efficient bit of MAFF.

Wednesday 21st March 11.30 p.m. The worst day so far and I am in absolute despair. The little ping my computer gives off when emails come in now sounds like an echosounder in a submarine, ping, ping, ping, ping, each one telling me of more cattle and sheep flocks hit by the disease.

There is an emergency debate today. I go into the Chamber at 3.30. I cannot bear to hear Blair say that everything is under control so I avoid PM's Questions. I would get so angry I would be expelled and the Speaker has already ticked me off. I have so much to say, so much irritation at the bungling of this, that I will never do it in the time. Where do I start and how do I present my latest rescue plan? In the end I thought my speech was rubbish and I never reached my peroration. Colleagues were kind and said it was brilliant but they always say that, just to be nice.

I went into the Chamber with ideas for action and a belief that with more vets and soldiers we could make a difference and get on top of it, and now at 11.30 p.m. I know that all is lost. The sheer devastation contained in the emails from Christine means that in one day we have lost 7,000 cattle and 21,000 sheep. A few more days of that and nothing will be left.

Matt's son phones me. He, like everyone else, wants his sheep killed hoping it will save his cattle. I tell him I will argue for that since it is sensible but that he must prepare for the worst. His voice is completely flat. He says that mentally he has but he has not told the rest of the family yet. I end as usual by saying 'if there is anything I can do?' It sounds so bloody feeble!!

I prepare another fax to send to every vet in my constituency and every farming leader. It says, 'I desperately need advice on where we go from here. Is there anything more I can ask from the Government now that may make a difference quickly enough? I feel despair and have come to the conclusion that we have lost the northern half of our county'. I go on to ask them to consider a drastic 'firebreak vaccination' policy whereby we try to save the National herd and South Cumbria by cutting a belt from the Irish Sea to the Pennines, vaccinating everything inside it and then killing them later. An Armageddon scenario and how have we come to this when only last week we were still talking about saving most of our flocks?

One vet has just faxed me back and ended with the words, 'I am dried up of all emotion. I am very thankful for all your efforts and wish you all the strength God can give you.' I know that dried up feeling. Like a wet rag that has been wrung out.

But my final words on this are those of another vet who said, in echoes of the Kohima memorial, dedicated to those soldiers of the Kings Own Royal Border Regiment and all the others in the Forgotten Army who fought in Burma, 'David, if we have to do this, when it is all over tell them that to save the National Herd we have sacrificed Cumbria'.

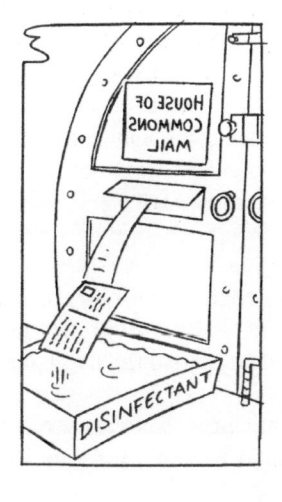

Anne Hopper

Anne Hopper was a member of staff at BBC Radio Cumbria's Barrow studios for twelve years before retirement. During the crisis she returned to the station to co-ordinate and present a foot and mouth information service.

Two years into retirement, which I always considered was premature anyway, and the call came: 'We've probably got more work than you'll want to handle'! That was the first indication I had that foot and mouth disease had arrived in Cumbria, and I was to take charge of the dispensing of information to all who needed to know the up to date position every day. Seven days a week and 12 hour shifts in the early-to-mid dark days of the outbreak. Bearing in mind the service was aimed at those in the agriculture industry, we began with five minute bulletins at five to the hour, just ahead of the regular news bulletins seven times a day from breakfast through to supper time.

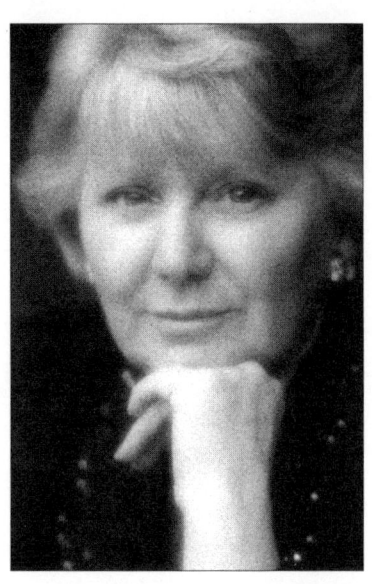

Photo: Tina Luke Sepias

As well as getting details of infected farms, animals involved and geographical areas, I keep an up to date record of numbers of cases, locally and nationally (which has actually proved very useful for the Ministry from time to time!) Systems were put in place to record schools closing because of local culls, events cancelled, and help, support and advice is available for those affected. Regular updates are sent to England Online, our BBC web site compilers, to keep those with Internet access up to date, especially valuable in a county where radio and TV signals are non-existent in some areas.

Life is one big learning curve, it's said, and I certainly didn't expect to add to my meagre knowledge of farming practices, disease symptoms, visitor figures and official statistics, not to mention trying to unravel statements like 'the dagging of hefted flocks'. Excuse me? (that's said in the American way!)

This particular learning curve was very steep because so many people were relying on BBC Radio Cumbria for vital information that it seemed impossible to get from anywhere else, let alone from the people who should have been supplying it, i.e. the Ministry, which I soon learned to call MAFF until it became DEFRA. See what I mean? It's another world! That the people who should have known better were taken as much by surprise by this outbreak as anyone else was the first shock - one of many I would be treated to in the coming weeks - so it was necessary to establish a working rapport with the people who *had* the information I wanted to pass on to those who *needed* it - the county's farming families.

They needed to know where the disease had been confirmed, and whose farm had gone down; was it a neighbour, a friend, a relation? And as I sat before the microphone each day, with the list of cases mounting, I felt so helpless. I know I *was* helping, because when people couldn't get information from official sources, they would phone me - and months later they still are. They ring with bottled up frustration almost before I've closed the microphone, ready for a coffee, the anger spilling over, often followed by the tears and an apology. None is needed. Often their need is just to have someone to talk to, who might be able to help, and if anyone has any doubt about where the BBC stands in people's esteem, even today, you should have been with me over the past few months. With the practical work done in the allotted time, the day frequently extended from 6 a.m. well into the evening, telephone clamped to my right ear. Could I find out about this, about that, *we* can't get any information!

But we *did* get the information (I like to think that after mutual suspicions were overcome MAFF/DEFRA and I reached a mutual understanding) and we dispensed it as rapidly as we could, and absorbed what came back to us: the cries of anger, of despair, of livelihoods ruined, of bewilderment that no one seemed then, and even now, half a year later, to know what to do to stop the remorseless spread of this dreadful virus.

I haven't had the experiences of some of our reporters who had to visit the slaughter and burial sites in the early days when, thank God, the killing was more public than it is now. It needed to be, so that people could see what went on. I felt for them, and I don't think I would have coped as well as they seem to have done. Farmers, men as well as women, young people whose whole lives have been spent on their farms, have cried down the phone to me. I've listened. And then I've cried afterwards - but if you don't witness something first hand the impact isn't quite so devastating. And there's always that professional detachment to maintain - compiling and presenting the bulletins isn't a problem – but it's a different story afterwards when the realisation comes that your words have meant misery and ruin for many, many people.

08.55 script   Duration: 4'38"

Foot and mouth Bulletin Script for: 8.55 am - Saturday 31st March 2001

Fifteen new cases of foot and mouth in Cumbria have been confirmed by the Ministry overnight - MAFF's total number of cases in the county is now three hundred and twenty-three. (323) The national total is eight hundred and thirty cases. (830)

The fifteen cases confirmed overnight are at:

Home Farm, Glassonby, Penrith
Marina House, Allonby, Maryport
Lower Dyke Farm, Calthwaite
Lesson Hall, Wigton
The Bow, Great Orton, Carlisle
Low How Gill, Milburn, Penrith
Dob Cross Hall, Gaitskill, Dalston
Howes Farm, Calthwaite
Dockray Farm, Wigton
Barrock End Farm, Armthwaite
East Farm, Newtown, Silloth
Stone House Farm, Seaville, Silloth
Glebe Farm, Kirkland, Penrith
Park House Farm, West Woodside, Wigton
High Flowery Hirst with animals at Birch Bush, Roweltown

The Ministry has today issued urgent advice for farmers on protecting cattle from foot and mouth. It says farmers should keep cattle housed as long as possible, do not graze cattle and sheep together - do not graze cattle in fields next to sheep.
And keep hill sheep on the hill - don't bring them in for lambing unless there is a disease risk on the hill. Next week MAFF hopes to expand on this general advice, and details will be posted on its website. We'll also bring you those details as soon as we're notified of them.   The MAF helpline can be of assistance if you have any queries - 0845 050 4141.

I've had several calls this morning about just where the uninfected area of the county now is - and whether or not farmers can still get licences to move their livestock to slaughter from that area.   The answer to that last question is yes - but licences are not issued at the weekend - the office will re-open at nine oclock on Monday morning ... this is the county's uninfected area as defined by

Printed:31/03/2001
11:16   by Anne Hopper   Page 1

And there are the animals, the lifeblood of the livestock farming industry, killed sometimes before being born, reduced to a stream of statistics by bureaucrats far away from the killing fields, simply because humans are at the top of the food chain and it's not considered necessary to treat the animals with the respect that I feel they deserve. They serve us, they provide our food, and I believe we owe them more than we've given them. Professional detachment gone again!

That's been my learning curve, a practical one and an emotional one. I've learned a lot in the past few months. I fear this outbreak isn't anywhere near being over yet, that it will go on after I've ceased to be directly involved. Today there are the farmers who are still desperately hoping that the virus won't reach their herds and flocks, who hang on to every word of the bulletins I read, knowing that if their neighbour's farm has been infected, it could be their turn next though they've survived thus far.

I've been privileged to help, if the dispensing of devastating information can be said to be helpful, and if I have one hope, it is that we learn from this dreadful experience, and never allow anything like this to happen again.

Written on 13 August 2001. Four more cases in Cumbria have been confirmed today. And we have just learned that 3.75 million animals have been slaughtered on infected premises nation-wide ..... and yet we read in the national press that the crisis is over!

NO ENTRY: Animal Disease Control Precautions

Maggie Norton

Maggie Norton is a writer and story-teller who lives in Ulverston.

I'm commissioned to support the testimonies of anyone affected by foot and mouth disease, become a non-political observer, and write poems that rise out of the meetings with those affected. I've met hill-farmers who have lost their stock, guesthouse owners, ministers, smallholders, rare-breed farmers and families living in dread.

If tourism is the golden thread that runs through our economy, then the canvas is a homespun cloth of farming families and dependant traders that underlies the social structure. I have felt privileged to see through windows opened onto courage, resourcefulness, neighbourliness, frustration, despair, anger and grief. I've been made so welcome. 'Yes, tell it like it is. Let's learn from our troubles. I want my story to be told. Let's know how to deal with it next time.'

As for the poems I write, what form should the works take? Free-verse? Traditional forms? Should I reach for rhyme? Perhaps a poem about each person I met? A figure in the landscape, a monologue in a particular voice, a narrative? Potent images emerged in five-line poems; a sonnet about a dale wrote itself; a long poem about a rare-breed farmer fell into rhyming couplets, and from somewhere a badger talks to a vixen.

The poem that follows came from a meeting with a farmer called Peggie who phoned Alan Smith on BBC Radio Cumbria with an angry response to Tom, a previous caller.

Peggie in the Duddon Valley

Oh I'd such emotion, there was no put-on.
It came right from where it should have come.
'Can you hear me Alan?' I said.
'Loud and clear', and that's all comment he med.

'Now Tom', I cries, 'I'm that sorry you spoke!
Your next piece of lamb, I hope you'll choke!'

I can picture it now, at what I said
when I picture his face turning red
for I bet his wife said,'Oh Tom, why ever,
why did you ring Radio Cumbria!'

We're that sorry for hill-farm lads and lasses.
They're a special breed of folk.
                                           If they passes
They won't be replaced when this is over.
Our way of life will be slipped between covers
Of books and films.

Like our hefted sheep we're bred to the fell
and doesn't this bonny valley show how well
we manage our stock?

And my phone never stopped. So many'd heard.
They said, 'we'd tears when you spoke them words
from your heart! We'd no idea.
Our prayers go with you and your fear
For the stock in the valley. May they be spared'.

Like my dad used to say, 'we're here to share
whatever we have in this wonderful world'.

Whatever we have it's only held
one for another. We must conserve
as well as we can, as God preserves
us and holds us up in his hand
and folk like Tom must understand
how folk like us work with the land.

Sarah Beattie

Many young people and children have been affected by the foot and mouth outbreak. Sarah Beattie who lives near Dalston and attends Caldew School is one of them.

My name is Sarah Beattie. I am 15 years old and I have a brother, Tom, who is 12. My parents farm Brackenhow Farm near Bridge End which is a 200 acre dairy farm. Our dairy herd and young stock got foot and mouth and were slaughtered on the 19th April 2001, a day which will not be forgotten because of the terrible effect which it had on my family, and also that day is my mum's birthday. When I heard that our neighbour's farm had been confirmed, I was really upset because I realised that we could be next. So as we didn't miss any school my brother and I were sent to stay at our grandparents' who live opposite our school. At the weekends we went to our gran's in Carlisle with our cousins who were also affected by foot and mouth. This was very upsetting and disruptive. I was taking exams at school, and it was difficult to concentrate on revising. We were at my gran's house when my auntie's farm was confirmed with foot and mouth. We were all crying and comforted each other. I still hoped we would escape this disaster.

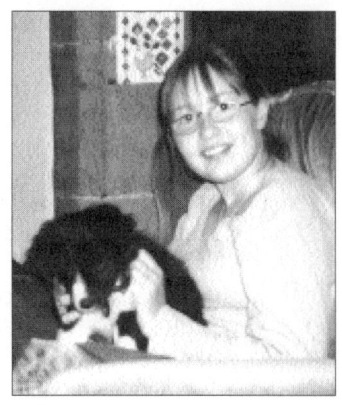

We were away for two weeks and came home for the Easter holidays. I thought we were going to make it as there hadn't been a case near us for 10 days. On 18th of April I was at a friend's house when my mum phoned to say we had F & M. I was numb and didn't know what to feel. Thoughts were flying though my mind, but I was with some really great friends. I couldn't go home until it was all over so I went to stay with my friend Melissa. My brother went to stay at my gran's as he didn't want to be at the farm when the animals were destroyed. He found the situation very distressing. Even now he doesn't want to talk about it and told gran he would try to think we had sold them so he wouldn't have to think about what had really happened. Going home on the Sunday afternoon was very strange. The farm was so quiet with no animals, just empty sheds. It has been hard for my dad and granda; they are used to getting up at 5.30 a.m. every morning but now there is nothing to get up for.

While this has had a devastating effect on us, it has brought the family together more with my dad not working such long days and having more time for family life.

Marje Thomlinson

Marje Thomlinson worked as an Administration Assistant at Caldew School in Dalston during the foot and mouth outbreak. She wrote this account of how the school was affected at the beginning of May.

The first declaration of foot and mouth brought with it memories of the 1960s outbreak when as a teenager the only impact on my life was the cancellation of the RAC Rally of Great Britain.

The 2001 outbreak turned my world upside down. I live and work in a rural community and at the outset would never have imagined how this virus would affect the day to day life of someone not directly connected with farming.

I work in Reception at Caldew School, Dalston, a rural secondary school which draws the majority of its pupils from a catchment area ranging from the Eden Valley to the Caldbeck fells, the marshes of Burgh by Sands to the outskirts of Carlisle racecourse. One of our GCSE courses is in agriculture and the school has a unit which rears pigs, cattle, sheep and poultry and this is a strong part of the school's identity. The birth of a new litter of piglets is always greeted with interest and the lambs are just part of our school as they graze in their adjoining field. I live in Stockdalewath, a farming hamlet and what remains of my husband's family are still farmers.

It soon became obvious that the school was going to be badly affected by the out-

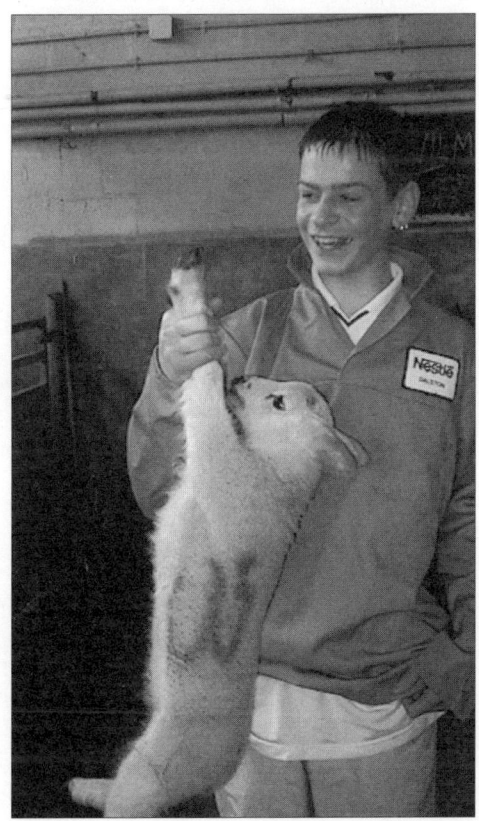

Pupil Alan Steel with one of the school's lambs

break. Our first call came from the Armathwaite area. Their child would not be in school today as they had been served with a D-Notice as they had a suspect animal. Call after call followed that day from worried parents who saw their farming livelihood threatened. At first there was a vacuum but soon the local education authority came up with guidelines for us to follow and for the first two days we found ourselves repeating them time after time. Then the goal posts changed, the advice was different, so we learned the new rules and again repeated them. As we spoke to parents we became a 'listening ear'. They were frightened, isolated, distraught. We shared it with them hoping in some way that just by talking with them it would help because we felt so helpless ourselves that we couldn't do more. They were a barometer, often warning us of a new outbreak before it came into the public domain.

Radio Cumbria was a godsend. Each morning I listened to the ever growing list of confirmed cases and on going into school discussed it with my colleagues. We were bombarded at every turn, parents, radio, TV, staff and pupils. By this time we had between 30 and 40 children not attending school. The LEA was most understanding and dictated that even if a child did not live on an infected farm, if the parents wished to keep the child at home, they would mark their absence as authorised. We got work together for them and either posted it or arranged for it to be dropped at their farm gate.

The school management paid lip service at first simply posting notices and putting a bit of straw near the astro turf entrance, but no other precautions were taken. The crisis deepened and our Chair of Governors, a farmer herself, threatened to resign unless we put down some disinfectant mats. This concentrated the mind and the mats were provided. Advice was sought on disinfectant strengths for vehicles etc. and otherwise we tried to carry on as normally as possible. The Internet and MAFF web sites were frequently referred to and provided much valuable information and advice.

Then came the black day. A call to a parent was answered with sobbing, she was deeply distraught but managed to tell me that they were going to slaughter all the animals in a 3 km radius. They were going to be ruined and her healthy stock would all have to go. I put the phone down and sat there stunned - all my neighbours, family and friends would lose everything. The tears flowed and I felt a comforting arm round my shoulders. My colleague too lived in a badly affected area and when I told her what was going to happen she too cried as the full implications of the new policy sank in. It was a miserable day for us all. That night I phoned or wrote to every person I knew who was affected by this just to let them know they weren't alone and I was thinking of them. I was glad to receive calls and emails from friends in other parts of the country asking how things were affecting us.

Later that evening a clarification of government policy brought a welcome uplift. Cattle were not to be slaughtered in the 3 km cull.

The ever increasing piles of rotting carcasses met you at every turn as you came into school. The smell of burning pyres permeated our classrooms. But what of our animals? So far so good, they were healthy, but the 3 km cull would take them all. Negotiations were in hand to make sure that the animals were not slaughtered at the school premises and they would be cremated on a nearby fire. Information came from a reliable source that this fire would not take place as Nestlé, which has a large plant next to the school, had taken it right to Downing Street to stop the fire as the smoke would go into their factory. The animals stayed and the pyre was dismantled.

We prayed that the animals would not get foot and mouth because if they did the school might have to be shut for 6 weeks, a nightmare with exams coming up. This further sharpened the management's actions and the whole agriculture block was closed off so no one could get anywhere near it. Twice the vet came because a pig was not well and I was aware of a churning deep in the pit of my stomach, but both times they were false alarms. The school became the centre of media attention. I saw the resulting coverage on the TV

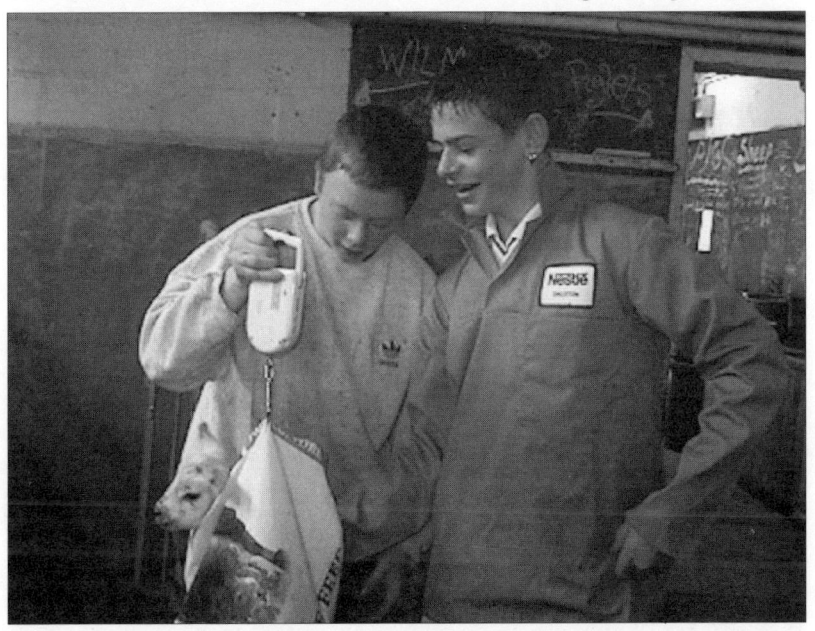

Pupils Alan Steel and Jason Haworth weighing lambs in the school agricultural unit

and heard it on the radio and was very proud of our head teacher and pupils for the excellent manner in which they represented the school.

Still the day to day pressure continued of calls from parents. We felt ground down by it all but realised how little our pressure was when compared with what was being suffered by our farming parents and friends. It was hard to watch grown men cry and to share with mothers their experiences of the actual events as they unfolded. They needed to talk, so we listened and hoped we were helping.

We could still be moved to tears – Peter Frost-Pennington's poem was taken from the Radio Cumbria web site and his agony was there for all to see. We heard horrible tales on the Radio Cumbria nightly phone-in and many farming friends related how their cattle had suffered with the disease: tongues falling out, ulcerated udders, terrible feet and the sheer speed with which it had spread through their herd, sometimes in a matter of a couple of hours. It was like a horror film which just kept repeating. They all paid tribute to the army personnel, their efficiency and patience, yet the sight of their Land Rover at a farm gate still brought a sinking feeling as you passed by - it was like the tolling of the lepers' bell - unclean - yet another farm had become infected.

Our school facilities were also affected. Events taking place at the school were cancelled by their organisers. Our Letting's Manager continually took calls asking if we were open. We were in the middle of having new buildings erected and the contractors were badly affected by the measures we had to put into place, but everyone pulled together to keep an air of normality for the pupils' sake.

Our first pupil came back. She seemed fine at first but later that day a small incident was enough to tip the scales and she became very upset. I am also a First Aider and together with another First Aider, we sat and talked her through it until she calmed down. She told us how badly she'd been affected by it all and she was particularly upset because her cat had gone missing when they'd let it out of the barn after the slaughter men had gone. LEA guidance has been issued on how to treat and help these children and we fully expect the effects to last for many months to come.

At Easter the school closed down and we went away on holiday. There was one field of lambs left between my home and work and on the last day before we left I mentally said goodbye because I knew I wouldn't see them again. How true this was because as we returned from holiday we left the motorway at Penrith and on the journey to Stockdalewath saw two ponies and one donkey. The fields were all empty and still the fires burned. The first phone call revealed that our last unaffected relatives had succumbed to the disease early that week - this meant with two exceptions, that every farming person we knew had lost their stock.

At school on Monday morning it was with relief that I heard our animals had been slaughtered over the holiday. Pressure had been brought to bear by the Director of Education to make sure that our cull took place during the Easter break. The pens and fields were empty.

Many children were now back at school; virtually everyone in our catchment area who could get the disease had got it, there was no one left to catch it. We still have about 10 children off at the end of April. Special dispensation has been granted to pupils affected by foot and mouth with regard to coursework deadlines for GCSE. It remains to be seen how the actual exams will be affected.

We are still taking calls and now the topic has changed to the disinfection procedures and how long and complicated they are. People are disorientated, lost and tell us how hard it is to get out of bed in the morning when there is nothing to get up for. The depression is obvious and also the fear of what the forthcoming months will bring to their income and life.

Things are quietening down at the beginning of May and life is starting to get back to normal when the sting comes in the end of the tale. One bright morning I opened the blinds to see an army Land Rover parked outside. The smallholding opposite me had the virus. During the course of the morning the 35 cattle were slaughtered, picked up by the grab, disinfected and loaded onto the wagon. The operation was quick and efficient and the team had gone

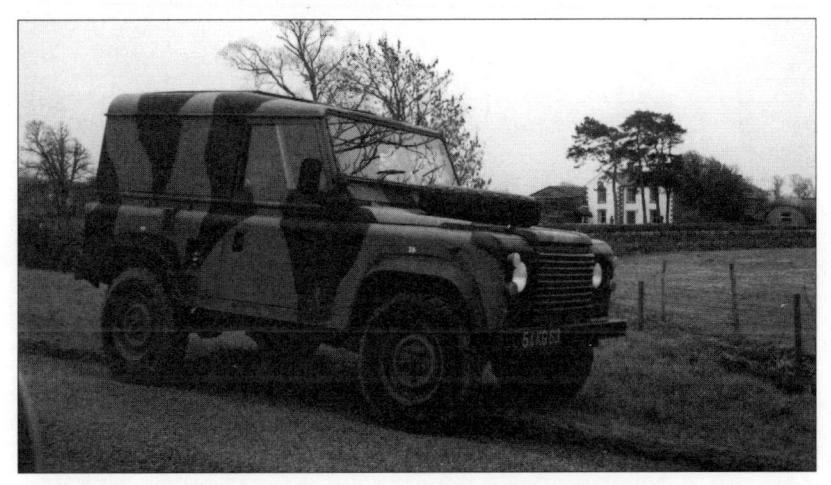

Army Land Rovers became a dreaded sight on the county's roads.

by lunchtime. Apart from the notice on the gate nothing remains to show that the killing fields had come so near to me, a far cry from the distressing scenes at the start of the outbreak.

Cases are still reported each day and some of these are our school children, but our list of children off school is now down to four or five. Some have not been at school for more than 10 weeks and this is particularly worrying, but regular contact with parents reveals it is their anxiety which is keeping the children away; they are terrified that the disease will still come to them and have sealed themselves off from the outside world. Our agriculture unit is still closed and will remain so for many weeks. MAFF have advised us that we will have to be disinfected even though our animals did not have the disease so the disinfectant team is awaited.

I have nothing but admiration for the vets, slaughter men, drivers, animal handlers, workers at Great Orton, office workers and officials at MAFF and the NFU, and our gallant army men, plucked from their normal work to administrate the logistics. They all deserve a medal.

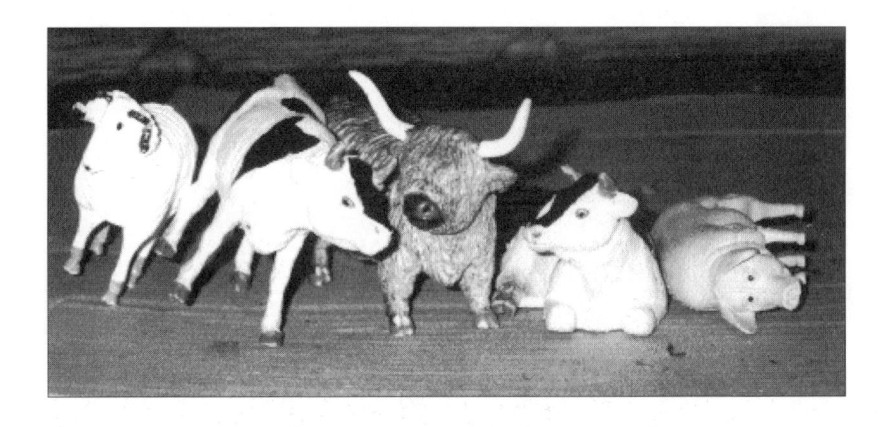

June Terry

June Terry lives in Blindcrake near Cockermouth with her three children, Philippa, Joshua and Alice. They have many farming friends and neighbours. June works in Keswick and the children attend schools in Keswick.

Our initial feelings when we first heard the news bulletins about the outbreak were ones of sheer shock and all we spoke to felt simply stunned. We listened to BBC Radio Cumbria at every opportunity.

Initially most of the cases were in Penrith and Carlisle but as time went on they became closer and closer until eventually there was a case at Bridekirk just down the road. We heard how farmers' livestock had been slaughtered and left in rotting piles for days. How awful it must have been for everyone involved, especially the kids. The 10 'til midnight phone-in on Radio Cumbria was often heartbreaking. What on earth could we do to help? I told the children, 'Just be ready to help in any way if you're asked.'

We made up our mind to have an open house for anyone wanting to stay. We often have kids from the village in and sleepovers so this was a way we could all help.

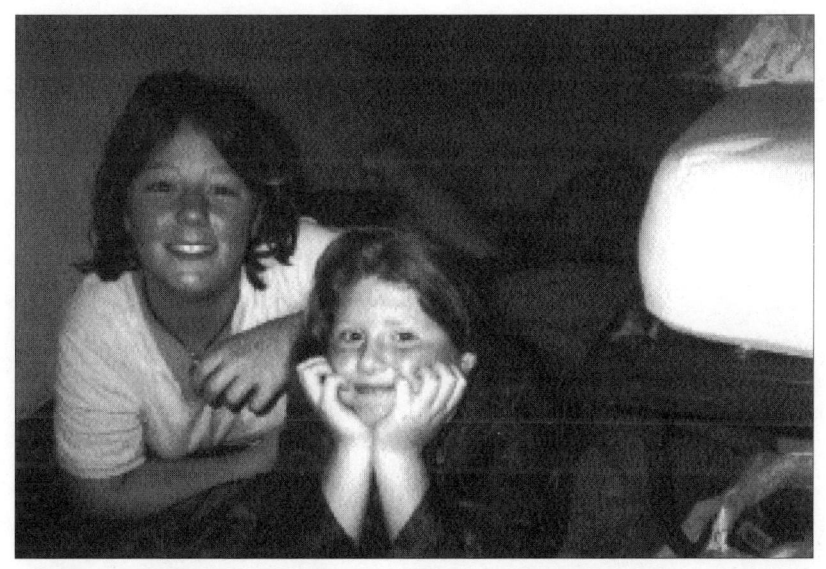

Pippa and Vicki, two of the sleepover kids with their sleeping bags.

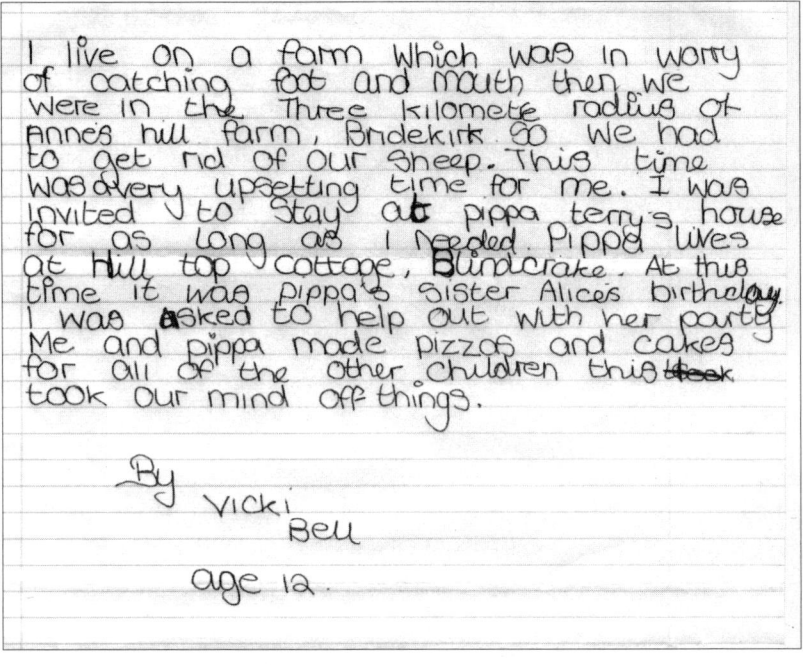

> I live on a farm which was in worry of catching foot and mouth then we were in the three kilometre radius of Annes hill farm, Bridekirk so we had to get rid of our sheep. This time was a very upsetting time for me. I was invited to stay at pippa terry's house for as long as I needed. Pippa lives at Hill top cottage, Blindcrake. At this time it was pippa's sister Alices birthday. I was asked to help out with her party. Me and pippa made pizzas and cakes for all of the other children this took our mind off things.
>
> By Vicki Bell
> age 12.

Needless to say, over Easter at the height of the worry we had a housefull. Every night. We played games like Monopoly. We played cards, painted by numbers and of course watched lots of TV and videos. At one time there were a dozen kids on one sofa bed!

We talked about foot and mouth and covered just about everything. Sharing worries made it easier. Many of these kids lived on farms and as the weeks and months went by I think the strain of it all was really beginning to show. All the lanes were out of bounds so you couldn't easily go for a walk or a cycle ride.

The case at Bridekirk was a real blow. This would mean that our friends, the Bells at Redmain, would lose their sheep. Would it mean Blindcrake too? We didn't know. Nobody seemed to know. Were we within three kilometres? Would the school bus still come? Trinity School in Keswick, where both Josh and Alice went, had given us a letter advising 'no children to work with livestock'. This really upset Josh because he had, until foot and mouth, helped on a local farm every weekend.

We had been using the main road to Keswick to avoid country lanes until someone pointed out that as the school bus still went that way there was no point in going the long way around.

Then, first day back at school, we noticed what looked like a ministry vet at Isel. We hoped it was just a precaution.

On our return from school that day we were waved round a tractor in the road and realised that we were following an army Land Rover. What came next was a really horrible experience. Around the next bend were all the tipper trucks, and men in white overalls spraying them down. In a field two men were slaughtering the most beautiful Herdwicks and piling them up against the fence. We were just stunned. Those in the car who weren't crying were silent. Where could we go? We couldn't go forward. We couldn't go back. We were trapped watching this terrible scene. It was just awful. Every day on our way to school we had admired the beautiful animals on this farm. Words couldn't describe how we felt. How on earth must the farmers be feeling?

Thankfully the next day they were gone, though the fields were like a battlefield. No sign of life anywhere and a feeling of death in the air. On our return we passed another field on the Blindcrake side of the river with one large pile of dead ewes and next to them a smaller pile of dead lambs. In another field there was a pile of young black Herdwicks.

2nd May – We've just arrived home to hear that our good friends the Clarkes have foot and mouth. We are all devastated. A lovely young family devoted to their animals. What must they be going through? Josh says he thinks he saw two MAFF men on the Clarke's quad bike up the back lonning. I rang to offer help. Neither of us could speak through the tears.

Now it's early June. It's been a horrid time for everyone. My friends are selling their B and B in Keswick, we're in the middle of an election and the Clarkes have been told their results were negative. They have lost all their stock, the village has lost all its sheep and lambs and more cases are being confirmed every day. God help us.

NO ENTRY: Animal Disease Control Precautions

Trevor Hebdon

Trevor Hebdon is Chief Executive of Harrison and Hetherington Ltd, operators of Borderway Mart, Carlisle, the largest livestock auction mart in Europe.

In terms of life changing moments, the announcement which I heard on BBC Radio 4's Today programme on the early morning of that fateful day in February must have registered very highly on my personal scale of 1 to 10. The discovery of foot and mouth disease in some pigs at an abattoir in Essex seemed to me far off, and I could not have imagined the length and depth of the devastation which was to befall Cumbria.

Within hours of the announcement Borderway Mart at Carlisle was totally shut down and at the time of writing (August), sales of livestock through our rings remain a distant memory as the tail of foot and mouth persists in our county and so many uncertainties prevail as to how the future shape of our farmstock business will look. When will we know what the new normality will be?

The buzz had gone out of Borderway, snuffed out like a candle – the mart's car parks empty of farmers and their vehicles, the unloading docks empty of drivers and their wagons and trailers, the alleyways and pens empty of yardsmen and the livestock they handled, the rings empty of auctioneers

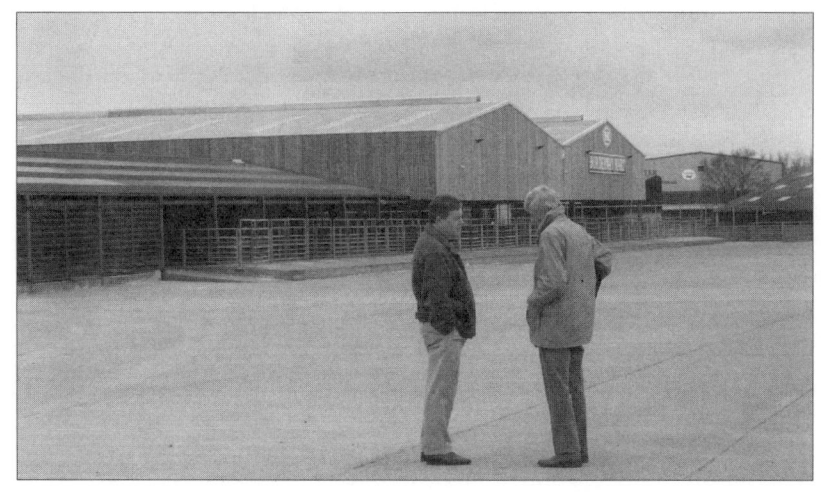

Trevor Hebdon, left, and Harrison and Hetherington Chairman Ian Walker in an unnaturally empty Borderway.

and their vendors and buyers together with the livestock they were trading, the offices empty of clerks and their customers and the concourse and cafeteria empty of the mart crack. When will the distinctive, and sorely missed, sights, sounds and smells of Borderway return?

Every Monday alone we would handle upwards of 2,500 cattle and 6,000 sheep, every Wednesday and Friday more cattle and sheep – and in the peak seasons, we would be selling at Borderway six days per week, commercial and pedigree livestock across five sale rings from dawn till dusk, with the cleansing of the mart and the office work continuing into the night long after the last fall of the auctioneer's hammer for the day. What is a mart without livestock?

From the diseased pigs at the abattoir in Essex foot and mouth was traced back to a farm in Northumberland, spreading like wildfire across north Cumbria and beyond – it was out of control before many realised with the catastrophic outcome of which we are all now too familiar.

Before the month of February was out we were drawn in to the heart of the crisis, making available a team of auctioneers to assist in the valuation of infected livestock prior to their slaughter. These were the most harrowing of times for our farming customers whom we knew so well and whose lives were in turmoil - and for our auctioneers for whom a typical day, at the height of the epidemic, might begin with arrival at the first infected farm at 6.00 in the morning and depending upon the numbers and complexity of the livestock, might involve visits to a further four farms in the same day in an attempt to keep ahead of the slaughter men and deal equitably with the valuation work in hand. Bio-security arrangements were an additional pressure with many of our auctioneers having their own livestock and being unable to return home, in some cases for up to nine weeks at a time.

And what of our other farmstock staff? A number, and in particular our part time yardsmen and office staff, were laid off at the outset as there was no work to do at the mart. I can remember vividly those early staff meetings, the anxieties, the frustrations and the unknowns. Others asked to be laid off to take up offers of outside work. Many agreed to remain on reduced salaries and wages and short time working. And we were fortunate to be able to out-source others to MAFF (DEFRA) to assist in the fight against this dreadful disease. Whilst they have all suffered grievously, their resilience and enduring spirit have been magnificent and a credit to them all.

It was late March when the army arrived, turning Rosehill into an emergency logistics centre overnight. At Borderway our open yard area, car parks and some of our offices were commandeered, strict bio-security measures implemented, Portakabins delivered, services installed, timber and

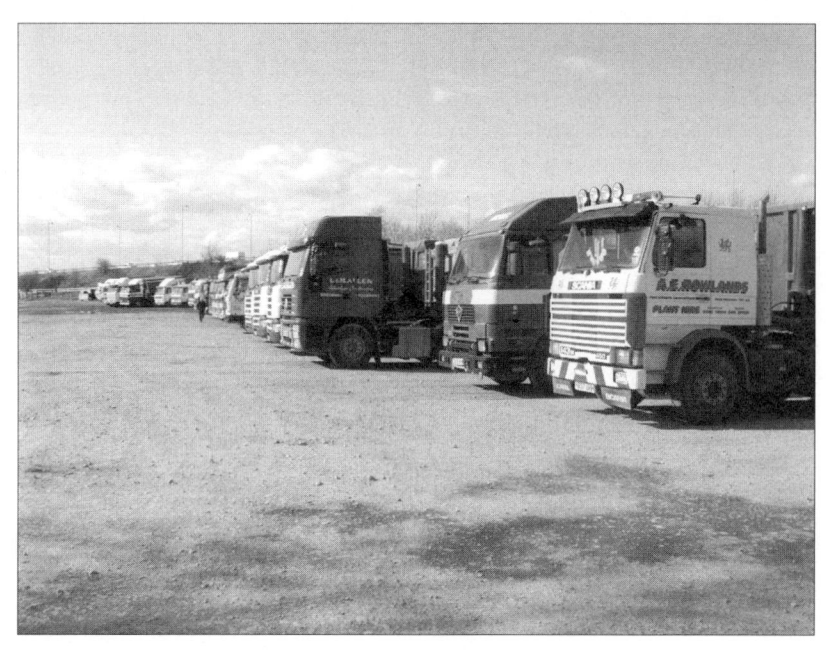

Carcass disposal lorries

coal stored for the pyres and vehicles and machinery of all types assembled to assist the army in its campaign. Late one evening, when that day's work was done, I can recall counting in excess of 140 carcass disposal wagons, 70 loaders/diggers and 40 disinfectant transit vans on site.

Not only have the events of the past six months deeply affected farming and the whole agricultural industry of which Borderway is an inextricable part, but also the entire fabric of Cumbria – no one has escaped, and it will be a long road to recovery. However, we must look to the future and here at Borderway, we are doing all we can to assist in getting Cumbria back farming as soon as we have rid ourselves of this dreadful disease and we can commence restocking in earnest. I will relish the day when Borderway is once again bursting at the seams with livestock.

NO ENTRY: Animal Disease Control Precautions

Jenny de Robeck

Jenny de Robeck lives with her husband and daughters near Sebergham between Wigton and Penrith. They're not farmers but their home adjoins farm buildings. On March 26th the cattle and sheep housed just a hundred yards from their front door were slaughtered after contracting foot and mouth. Jenny and her family were trapped at home for the eleven days it took for the carcasses to be removed. This is her diary.

Monday 26th March

There is no sound now. Every field is empty. Empty, empty, empty. The sheep lie dead beside the silage. The cattle lie dead in the yard at the top of the drive.

Tuesday 27th March

A light fall of snow in the night, and a bitter wind this morning. But the most horrific thing is the terrible silence. You could until yesterday hear the cows clanking and lowing and the sheep calling. Now there is just silence with the wind moaning round the front of the house. I find myself doing odd things. Baking, cleaning, ironing, restless, unsettled. The dogs and cats are clingy. For no reason at all I burst into tears.

The bodies of the cattle lie sprawled in the yard, bloating, heads outstretched, tongues hanging out, undignified. Just appalling. It is always a horrible experience seeing an animal 'down', a sight that makes you gasp and stops the heart beating, but to see a whole herd like that is just indescribable. It makes you want to vomit.

MAFF are coming tomorrow to spray disinfectant on the carcasses. No sign yet of them being moved.

Wednesday 28th March

The smell is quite horrendous. To go outside now, even into the garden with the cats and dogs is revolting. It is essential to wear a scarf round your face on account of the stench. The fridge gets emptier. Rosie is now emailing Tesco for grocery deliveries.

Thursday 29th March

Still nothing. Still confined. Still the smell. Still Blair waffles about an election. The Dept of Environment, which we have contacted re. health and rats, is not allowed to help. MAFF is useless. The army will not answer left messages. The stink seeps through the window frames, up plug holes, under doors. Lorries this p.m. They have come to remove the sheep. We are so cut off it's unimaginable.

Friday 30th March

Sunny. Stinky. Letter in the 'Daily Telegraph' and 'The Times' came to do an interview about the plight of the non-farmer hostaged by MAFF. They were supposed to come today to disinfect the cattle but no one has been. Poppy delivered some milk to the box at the road end tonight as we are getting low and, bless her, a box of chocolate eclairs. What a treat!

Saturday 31st March

Went down to the cattle grid to collect groceries from Pauline. We really do feel 'unclean', as if even touching someone beyond the boundary will contaminate them.

Sunday 1st April

A week now since the MAFF vet turned up on our doorstep. The cows are still here. Richard phoned and phoned MAFF and the army to no avail. After a dozen attempts R. gets the army who say that an extra 300 lorries are being brought into Cumbria today to cope with cattle carcasses, but we still don't have any idea when our fallen stock will be shifted.

Monday 2nd April

Blair still refuses to give a date for the election. The disinfecting people are here again, only the third time in 8 days. After badgering the army again R. learns that they are collecting stock culled on the Saturday before our Monday. Why couldn't we have been informed of this before? Why do we have to bludgeon it out of people? Is it a secret?? Being kept in the dark is much worse than knowing the truth.

Tuesday 3rd April

Still no news. Our supply problems are bad. Concocting ridiculous meals out of a scrap of ham, a cabbage and a pound of rice. But it must be a nightmare to have children around and burly farm folk to feed.

I went out, as I do each day, to check the carcasses were still there. You get such stupid ideas that perhaps the wagons came through the night and took them away. No. They are still here. As I write, at 11.40 a.m. I cannot see us ever being released from this hellish situation. The excuses we are given for no progress are quite unbelievable. Today, 'Sorry, all the lorries have all been sent to the Borders'. An hour later, great excitement! There's a chance we could see some wagons this afternoon. One hour later and it's all off again.

All this makes me very irritable and near to tears. R. has phoned a solicitor to enquire as to who he can sue for loss of earnings. I have not set foot outside this place since Friday March 23rd. That's eleven days.

Wednesday 4th April

A thick unbreathable pall of smoke now runs along the Caldew valley. So the stench of rotting carcasses is amalgamated with the stench of burning carcasses. The sun has disappeared. It is like the biblical prophecies about darkness covering the face of the earth. People keep phoning to see how we are, but I have to get them off the line as quickly as possible in case the army rings back. I have almost been rude to three people today.

All this, of course, makes you very paranoid. You begin to think MAFF and the army have a personal vendetta against you. It is just so depressing. David Maclean has just phoned. Apparently MAFF didn't pass our details on to the army so we are now one of 20 to 30 lots of people who have been waiting an eternity to have carcasses removed.

4.30 p.m. – We have just heard that wagons are on the way. Can you believe it, wagons are on the way!

5.20 p.m. – 8 lorries have arrived but no loaders.

5.45 p.m. – Our farmer, equipped with one tractor and bucket, has begun loading the first wagon. Real loaders eventually arrive. R. came in having spoken to the drivers. They are horrified at the carnage. The cattle on top were able to be lifted in one piece but the ones underneath were almost molten. The men had never seen anything like it. One of the drivers said that their fleet had sat idle in a lay-by for three hours while MAFF decided where they should go. Another told of how he'd arrived at Great Orton fully loaded with carcasses and discovered he'd been given the wrong paperwork. He had to take his load back to the farm it had come from. Another had lost a whole day's work because the loaders weren't co-ordinated with the lorries.

7.45 p.m. – Lorries still here. You know, we all felt that when this moment arrived we'd be filled with an enormous sense of elation, but the opposite is actually true. We feel exhausted, emotional and nothing short of plain damn sad that those in power have let the country get to such a low. We have lived 100 yards from dead, rotting cattle for a full ten days.

I am going to bed shattered

Brigadier Alex Birtwistle

Brigadier Alex Birtwistle, OBE, MA, late Commander 42 (North West) Brigade, Colonel The Queen's Lancashire Regiment and Deputy Colonel The Lancastrian and Cumbrian Volunteers led the Army's support to MAFF in Cumbria, Lancashire, Greater Manchester and Merseyside for five weeks in March and April 2001. In gratitude for the support Cumbria gave him he has dictated this article.

On a Wednesday in the middle of March this year I got in the staff car to go north from Preston to Carlisle. It was to be a routine trip to visit a small detachment of some 20-30 regular and territorial soldiers, deployed under the command of the Chief of Staff of 42 North West Brigade, Major David Holt, to lend assistance to MAFF staff by showing them how to set up a simple operations room and by the provision of liaison officers on infected farms. I was within 10 days of finishing my term of duty, an event I was looking forward to enormously, not because I had not been conscious of the privilege of commanding the marvellous men and women in the Brigade but because in addition to being depressed I was physically exhausted after two and a half years of mainly nugatory work countering the adverse effects of successive divisional restructurings and the Strategic Defence Review. Nonetheless, on that day, heartened by the imminence of my retirement and bolstered by the many kindnesses shown to me on my various farewell visits, I settled down to attempt, as always, 'The Times' crossword having given instructions to my driver that if I fell asleep he was to wake me minutes short of Carlisle so I could read my brief.

He duly complied and, as I pulled into the industrial estate that held the

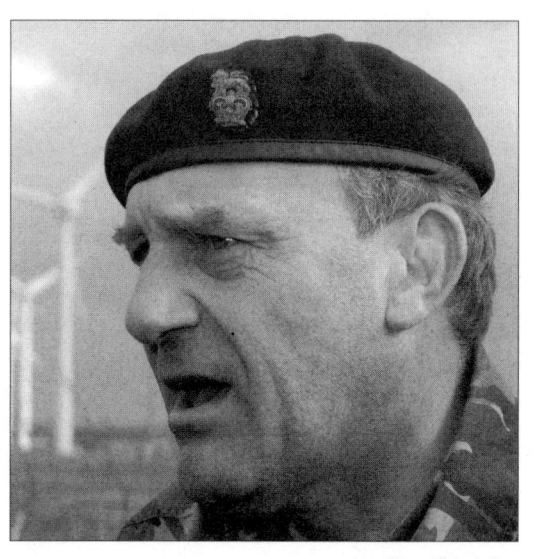

Photo: News & Star

MAFF offices, I anticipated nothing more than the pleasure of a customary 'meet and greet' and a hot cup of tea. And so it proved, but by the end of the day I had collected a number of points that I believed required my attention and had posed a couple of questions to the Chief of Staff about the future. We agreed we would speak on the telephone that night after 10.00 p.m. to resolve these issues.

I was still struggling with the crossword when he phoned just before 11.00 p.m. We concluded the business in hand and he then remarked casually, with what I thought was a slight frisson in his voice, that the Prime Minister was to make an unscheduled visit to Cumbria the following day. My inclination was, as always, to place confidence in him but some subconscious instinct caused me to ask, even though the military's involvement would be limited to a ceremonial handshake, whether he required my presence. He accepted the offer though I sensed he wished to spare me the trouble. He suggested that I arrive at 1.30 p.m. as the Prime Minister was due at 2.00 p.m. but I told him I would come a little earlier to prepare myself. Thus it was the next morning at 11.00 a.m. that I was once again disembarking in Carlisle with 'The Times' crossword, predictably yet again, incomplete. I knew from my previous experience of working to the Cabinet Office, under the previous administration at the time of the Bosnia hostage crisis, that if the Brigade was to become involved we were likely to have to operate in a politically charged atmosphere where many in Whitehall would feel uncomfortable to the point of paralysis working outside the normal parameters. Keen to put matters in order before I handed over to my successor in a few days time, and confident I could do so, I was nonetheless concerned that I knew nothing about the scale of the problem if there was to be an increase in activity. My worst fears were confirmed when the Chief of Staff remarked that the farmers had indicated that they were likely to request the proactive firebreak cull that they had stood out against some 10 days previously when visited by the Chief Vet. Knowing that it is best to get people to buy into the problem at an early stage I decided to produce a brief schematic of where the problems lay with the current operation and what would be required to upscale it.

Being by inclination and aptitude completely computer illiterate I asked David to procure me a typist. It was now about 11.30 a.m. and we were due to welcome the Prime Minister at 2.00 p.m. There then occurred one of those farcical episodes which, though totally trivial, remain vivid long after the memory of major events has passed. The Chief Clerk arrived bearing a laptop but had great difficulty in making it obey his instructions to split the page in half vertically and to produce a series of downward pointing arrows.

After 10 minutes of fruitless labour and repeated assurances that he would soon master the machinery, which he claimed no doubt truthfully to be suffering a minor and untypical lapse, I issued one of the few orders I have ever given in 33 years of military service and told him to forget it and to type as I dictated. We had already drawn up a list of the key points in the process from diagnosis to disposal and it merely remained to place those in the left hand column, linked subsequently by arrows drawn freehand and then photocopied, and to note in the right hand column the potential choke points at each of these stages of the operation. This we rapidly did. I sensed that both the Chief of Staff and the Chief Clerk doubted whether this document would ever be presented to anybody but, having been taught by my first platoon sergeant that foresight was not the thing on the end of a rifle, I took it with me intent on giving it to whomsoever would receive it if the opportunity arose. This proved fortunate for it was soon readily apparent that we were facing a potential shambles that was likely to grow into a major crisis.

The meeting convened around a number of circular tables pushed together in the upstairs room of the Auctioneers Arms adjacent to the MAFF complex. The Prime Minister and his Aides, local politicians, representatives of the local tourist industry, which nets four times what agriculture does in Cumbria, and of the farmers were there. Crucially it was the first time that I met my new boss, Mrs Jane Brown, a Senior Civil Servant 'parachuted' in from London to head the MAFF team. It was to be the second time I would work directly to a Senior Civil Servant in a crisis situation. On both occasions I have found it a pleasant and fruitful experience to work with first class brains at the interface between politics and the military.

As the meeting progressed with me, untypically, as a silent observer I reflected ironically on the days when Government policy was supposed to have been made in upstairs smoke-filled rooms over plates of sandwiches and warm beer. True, we had the sandwiches, though sadly no beer, but as my nicotine withdrawal symptoms and general impatience increased I could not help in thinking that, not withstanding the requirements of health and safety, it was a shame this Prime Minister did not smoke a pipe for I would then be able to have a cigarette.

After more discussions it became apparent that the farmers' wish for a cull would be met. It was at this stage the Prime Minister caught my eye and enquired of me, the sole uniformed figure in the room, whether the administrative arrangements in place would be sufficient to accommodate the upscale in activity predicted. Though not a logistician I had taken the guidance of my quartermaster whilst in command. Therefore I replied that I feared they would not. The Prime Minister then intimated to the general gathering that this should pose no problem because he was determined that the matter should be resolved as quickly as possible and that the resources of the Nation would be deployed.

We then adjourned for coffee. The Prime Minister and I found ourselves in each other's company and after some conversation he enquired how long I thought it would take to solve the problem. Never a man to offer hostages to fortune, though in my naivety I had mentally set myself in the intervening minutes a target of a week, I replied that I did not know but that I would have the administrative arrangements in place by 'Tuesday week'. The Prime Minister raised an eyebrow and enquired why I had selected Tuesday week. I replied that I only had two clean shirts for I was due to hand over command on that day. In retrospect I regret for his sake and mine that I was not more conscious of the gravity of the occasion but occasionally I am overtaken by an irreverent desire to see the humorous side of events.

The meeting reconvened and when concluded the Prime Minister made a brief statement to the press after which I went thankfully for a cigarette. I made contact with Mrs Brown and her staff and briefed the Chief of Staff that we might be likely to receive some form of direction to assist more comprehensively in the operations in support of MAFF. At this stage we had nowhere to operate from except an elevated Portakabin occupied by some 15 MAFF personnel under the highly effective and dedicated eye of Captain John Mayo of the Duke of Wellington's Regiment who was holding his own against great odds whilst teaching all concerned how to run a joint agency operation. His task was not made any easier by the fact that the MAFF regions did not reflect those of any other government department and he was constantly receiving telephone calls from the north-east reporting infections there. These required him to fill out the details on paper and fax them back to the north-eastern regional office. The noise level in the insulated box was ear-piercing with 15 phones constantly ringing and personnel coming in and out to be updated on the map. This went on 16 hours a day without respite and although at the time I thought that the matter could have been better expedited, I now realise what an enormous achievement Captain Mayo and his team of military liaison officers had already made. So, in the absence of any office space and without a Land Rover, I was constrained to sit either in my staff car or to walk up and down the car park in a light drizzle analysing the problem in advance of meeting with the Chief of Staff when he returned from liaising with MAFF. I rapidly came to the conclusion that it was an essentially simple operation requiring us to pick objects up at A and deposit them at B. Knowing that the objects could be either alive or dead, I drew 2 circles on the back of a cigarette packet, placed a square where they met to represent the disposal site or sites at B and allied this to the previous analysis which I had given to Mr Alistair Campbell and the Prime Minister's Aide. Working on the principle of trusting no one I then made a list of what could possibly go wrong, cross-referenced this to the choke points we had established earlier in the day, and decided that I would give the professional logisticians in the Brigade a run for the Nation's money.

Therefore I handpicked a small team which included Lieutenant Colonel Paul Baker, the Regular Commanding Officer of 156 Transport Regiment Volunteers and Captain Charlie Parr, a recently commissioned master chef who had just returned from a voluntary tour of the Balkans and summoned them to be in Carlisle that Friday evening. They were, and Colonel Baker had the foresight to bring his training Major, whom he no doubt intended to do the hard work for him. I briefed them that there had been some discussion about 3 airfield sites and told them to leave at first light in the morning to check their suitability from the logistical standpoint and that I would ensure that the Environment Agency followed them up to examine the environmental requirements.

In retrospect it would have been better if the party had travelled together for it was difficult to receive their reports the next day on one mobile telephone, but at the time I had no idea who represented the Environment Agency and I felt it important to get matters underway.

Saturday proved to be a heartening day. I still had no idea of the size of the problem nor had I any transport resources, though Captain Charlie Parr was busy with the Yellow Pages acquiring what transport and lifters he could. Paul Baker and his team reported that the Great Orton site was eminently suitable and Dr John Marshall of the Environment Agency and his inspirational team confirmed that it met all their requirements. Most importantly, MAFF's purchasing agents in London had stayed on duty constantly to ensure we could liaise with our local valuers day or night and thus it was that, having begun the reconnaissance at 8.00 a.m. by 4.00 p.m. we had secured the lease from the 6 interested parties on the airfield and were in a position to begin preparing the site.

Concurrently with the reconnaissance I had hired from an authorised contractor two large bulldozers and guaranteed, as he was still working without a MAFF contract note, the deal on my personal handshake. Naturally I ensured that after the proper negotiations had taken place he received quickly a contract note for I did not have in loose cash the sum I had undertaken to find if necessary.

Thus it was, that having waited anxiously throughout Saturday night to

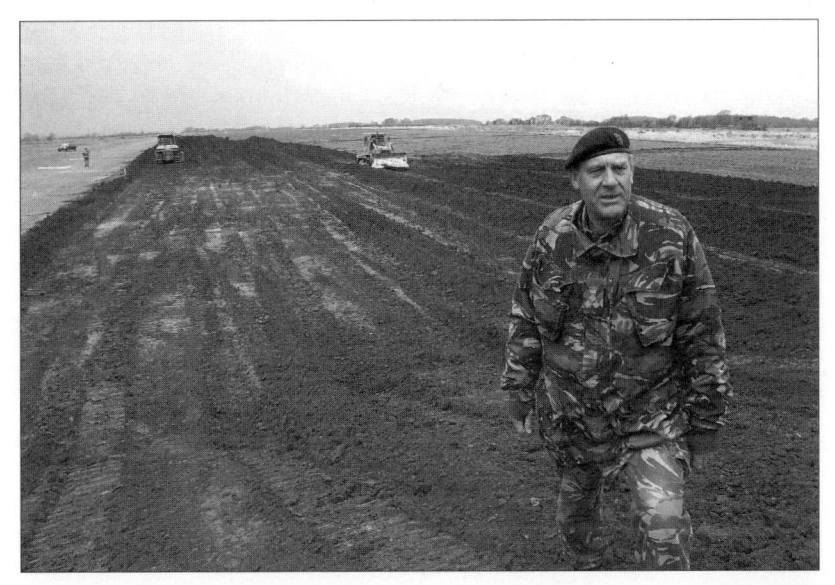

Photo: News & Star

meet the requirements of health and safety, we were able to start stripping off the first of 60 acres of topsoil at first light on Sunday morning, and by first light on the Monday morning we had nine spill-proof truckloads of sheep ready to dump. I was asked to delay the dumping so a press conference could take place and knowing that morale among the Cumbrian community was extremely depressed and, that it would take some time to shift the limited number of lifters we had from the first series of loading sites to the next and thus no time would in effect be lost, I concurred.

Until this operation began I had no experience of the media. True, on the Friday night I had been diverted into a car park in Penrith on my way home to do an interview for Lindsay Taylor of Channel 4. I had been extremely nervous but he was kind enough to stretch the truth sufficiently to say that I had done adequately and so the next morning I was slightly more confident when interviewed by John Humphries on the Today Programme. However, his opening question, 'Why wasn't the Army called in earlier - you're good at digging holes aren't you?' so astounded me that I let out an involuntary burst of laughter and no doubt caused the studio manager some concern for I was unable to respond for 5 or 6 seconds. Thereafter I realised that I could expect on some occasions a hostile ride and that mine and everyone's interest would probably be best served by accommodating the pressures on frontline journalists to give regular news updates to their editors. Therefore, I briefed them constantly on and off the record. Nonetheless I was still somewhat concerned when having done the collective press call with MAFF I was asked to do seven or eight down the line television interviews with all the major companies who had arranged their cameras at a 45 degree angle across the airfield from the first burial pit. However, the greatest fear is the fear of the unknown and by the time I had reached the fifth I was beginning to feel a little more relaxed.

In the days to come I was able to transfer more and more of the responsibility for briefing the press to my press minders. Drawn from the regular Army, the Territorial pool and the civil service they became firm friends and staunch allies but I made the point at the time that it was a shame that they had to be constantly changed for it took them a little while to read into the disease and be master of the background necessary to operate effectively in a politically charged atmosphere under the international press interest. At one stage we had 40 television crews outside Great Orton, several of them equipped with 120 ft cherry picker gantries capable of hearing our every word from miles away and of photographing our every move. It was therefore vital that nothing was said, deliberately or accidentally that would arouse criticism.

Later events were to demonstrate how a totally innocent and incongruous

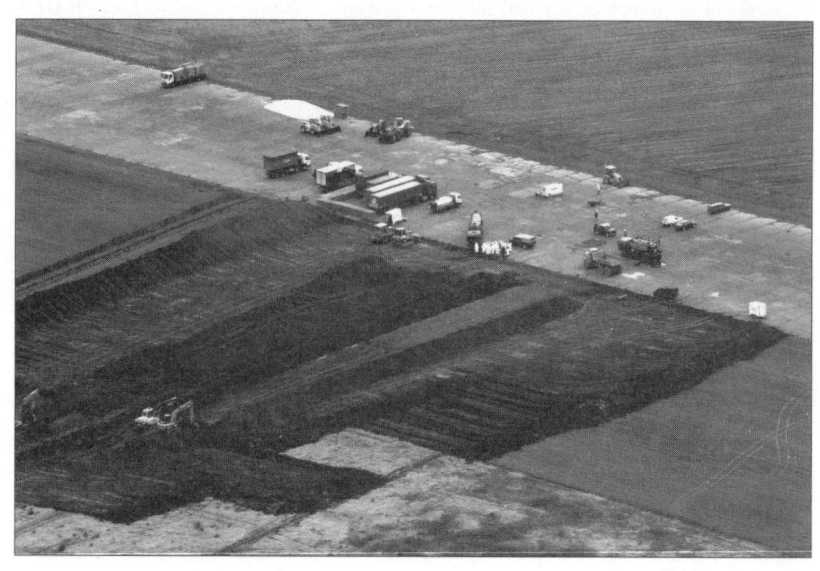

Photo: News & Star

Preparing the mass burial ground at Great Orton airfield

86

remark strictly in line with the MOD press line and government policy could be misinterpreted. Nonetheless, on the whole, our relations with the press were harmonious perhaps because we took the trouble to make ourselves available whenever we could, and mindful of the hospitality rules, spent our own money entertaining them late in the evening to brief them informally on the mechanistic problems we faced. I am pleased to say that many of them have written to me privately since and several of them keep in regular contact though we have an unwritten rule that we never speak about foot and mouth.

Within 2 or 3 days four ancient box bodies had arrived, immaculately maintained, from our local Territorial Signals Unit and these provided both a measure of shelter from the elements and refuge for me to lie down on the table and have a cup of tea and a cigarette as required. There was much talk at this stage of when the cull would begin and we were all amused to see many television journalists standing in front of the four box bodies implying to the world that these 4 vehicles would be the ones that undertook the logistical backup and that they would soon move from their present location to begin the disposal of one million animals. Their ignorance of the scale of events was shared by many others in and out of uniform. Indeed at one stage I thoroughly lost my temper with one of my colleagues in London, to whom I now apologise for I know from his subsequent performance and the reports I have received from many at DEFRA that, once he had worn himself into his webbing, he played a blinder.

From then on the operation increased in tempo and in volume. We appealed on TV, sometimes at hourly intervals, for the equipment we needed and concurrently began to gather the data that would enable me to carry out a further analysis of the problem.

I didn't conduct the formal military estimate: I wouldn't have known how to. In the fast moving situation clear analytical and lateral thought based on proven fact was sufficient and, anyway, my sense of irreverence would not have allowed me to complete the 'in order to' section in the standard format without disloyalty. One of the great things to realise in life is to know what one does not know and I realised very quickly that I knew very little about the disease. The listings of diseased dead animals were in chronological order and the census forms for live animals my instincts told me, having lived 25 years in sheep rearing areas, were likely to be inaccurate. I therefore decided to kill three birds with one stone, spare the over-stretched regular component, give employment to those TA and OTC personnel who could not go on summer camp, and publicise the flexibility of the Regional Brigade. I had already sent a Warning Order to all regulars to come to 12 hours notice to move and had added a paragraph that any territorial who wished to serve should consider himself or herself on the same notice, regardless of the fact I had been at that stage specifically prohibited by the MOD from deploying any TA personnel. Knowing the paralysis by analysis that was probably taking place I chose to interpret that order merely as not to formally mobilise and thus I accepted territorial volunteers from Day 1.

Concurrently, staff were working on the logistical problems posed by the two loops on the cigarette packet, later known as the testicular analysis, and in conjunction with MAFF and many other agencies had already set up controls for the first choke point, the process whereby live animals were to go on to the transport for eventual slaughter. This ensured that the slaughter site at Great Orton was not swamped by unscheduled arrivals.

The dead loop posed more problems. Because we were determined to do nothing without political guidance and the best scientific advice we waited what seemed an eternity for a disposal policy on cattle. This sentenced us to make double trips eventually. The central issue was what residual danger BSE posed and at up to what age, if at all, cattle could be buried. Here I made a fundamental mistake which was to come back to haunt me and potentially to bring the operation to a halt. On first briefing the press about the Great Orton site I had said that it offered not only the opportunity to bury safely but also to prepare, along the length of the entire runway, funeral pyres. I thought I had expressed myself with sufficient clarity but by accident or intent certain sections of the media chose to dramatise this simple logistic expedient by describing it as potentially the biggest bonfire of the century. Of course this was nonsense for it took £200,000 of material and three days to build a pyre sufficient to burn a mere 250 animals and we were faced with the prospect of disposing of a sum infinitely greater than this. However, it is possible that the potential social and political ramifications of such a bonfire, even though it were not physically possible, created a misappreciation in the minds of some outside Cumbria and we waited and waited for a clear policy to emerge.

Though worried by it, I was not at that time critical of the delay for, imperfect though the democratic process is, I did not wish to proceed without consent or authority. However I was conscious that if cattle as well as sheep had to be slaughtered on site, and this was an increasing possibility as we were approaching the time when they would be turned out from stalls, we would lose all we had gained both physically and in terms of morale.

Eventually a policy emerged: we were to bury those under 6 months, then under 3 years and finally on a Saturday lunchtime the Minister of Agriculture announced that cattle born after 1st August 1996 could be buried. I knew the burial capacity at Great Orton was finite and that if the disease spread we would soon be up against that limit. Incidentally I had been amused to see two qualified Chartered Surveyors attempting to work out how many square yards a certain number of sheep would fill and then engaging in a lengthy and totally serious debate about how to measure a sheep. I pointed out to them that I was merely a layman in their trade but if they knew how many sheep would go into a rectangular lorry they could perhaps work out how many lorries would go into a rectangular hole. It was interesting to see their expression of dismissive disbelief pass slowly into acceptance that I might have the germ of an idea.

However, back to the problem of cattle. Because we had always been led to believe that it would be necessary to burn them the great majority of those taking part had not considered it necessary to find fresh burial sites, merely to consider negotiating an extension of the Great Orton site on the assumption that there was as much land remaining we could use, as that we had already leased. Thankfully I did not place total reliance on this policy as it transpired parts of the extended Great Orton site were unsuitable for burial and of course because we were faced with a far greater problem in volume terms, of burying cattle once burning had been prohibited.

Serendipitously, a retired Territorial Army Officer had strolled into the operations room some days previously, dressed in an ageing combat kit smelling of moth balls and had announced that he was a civil waste disposal engineer who had called himself up to serve the Crown, the nation in general and myself in particular during the current crisis. He enquired whether I could use his services.

I put him on a seat, christened him Colonel Dumper to mirror my transport Lieutenant Colonel, Colonel Humper, and forbad him to sleep for 3 days. Armed with a telephone he was able to liaise directly and in the same technical terms with the ever helpful but exhausted staff of Cumbria Waste Management and, in conjunction with all the relevant environmental agencies, to begin negotiations to open the Hespin Wood site. This was a commercial landfill site already dug and lined with polythene and fitted with drains but without adequate access. After I refused the initial engineer's estimate of 10 days to make a tarmac access road they decided on a rough and ready solution taking 3 days, 10,000 tons of gravel aggregate, the insertion of the odd culvert here and there and about 600 metres of drainage pipes. To finish the job off they widened the existing stretch of access road to that point and five men and a woman laid a medium girder bridge in a night. Thereafter it was a simple matter of shipping in over 6,000 tons of domestic waste a day from Glasgow to put a 6 foot base lining across an area of some 400 metres by 200 metres to accommodate the first fleshy layer of an obscene lasagne. As a temporary expedient, whilst the works were in hand, we buried in the existing but almost full Hespin Wood domestic site.

By now we were some three and a half weeks into the operation and my staff who, after a quarantine period, had all taken a brief break at home, permitted me to go to St Bees for the day for a change of air. As I walked miles up and down the beach, the footpaths being of course closed, I received a succession of telephone calls, first from fairly important people in London but finally from Colonel Humper who informed me that he had just encountered serial 34 on the master events list of the exercise from hell: after all our efforts the Preston Police had proclaimed the major Hespin Wood tip to be the site of a murder enquiry and closed it forthwith. Tired and dispirited as I was I laughed at what I thought was a joke but Paul Baker assured me it was not. I told him I would ring the Chief Constable if necessary but he asked me to hold back, and thankfully, an hour later, I was informed that Colonel Dumper had pointed out that the two vehicles that had brought rubbish up from Preston were not equipped to have lifted wheelie bins and therefore neither the body nor the murder

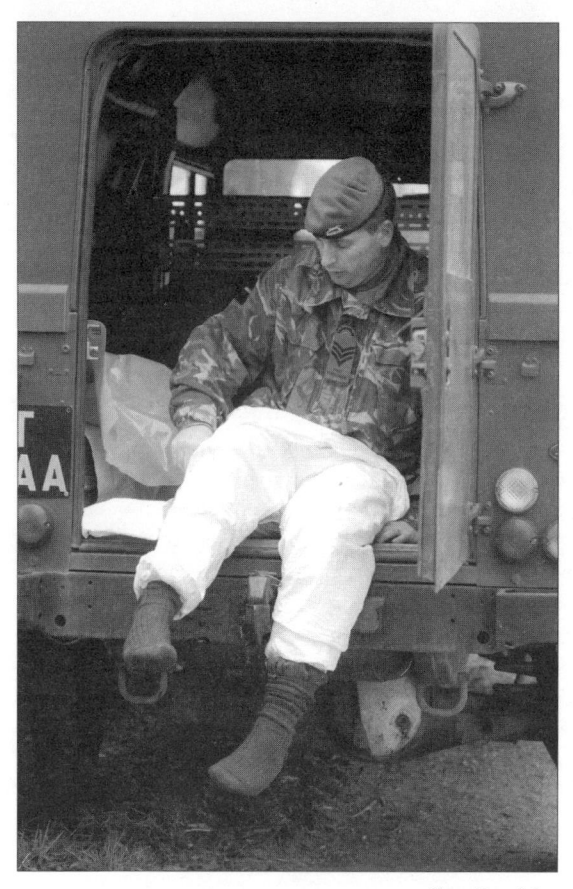

Photo: News & Star

Hundreds of army personnel were involved in the disposal of carcasses.

weapon could be in the waste. Thankfully this advice was accepted and operations soon restarted.

So overall, what conclusions do I draw from the operation? The first and overwhelming conclusion I draw is that the Army is much better than it gives itself credit for and it is a conclusion that I have since tested in civilian life. Others may disagree but I believe it to be the case for when our scratch team, many of them Territorials who changed at weekly intervals, arrived, the time from diagnosis to destruction was over 3 days. Yet within 6 days the time from diagnosis to complete disposal was, with one exception, always under 24 hours and on many occasions under 12 hours. This was a considerable achievement given that the countryside was littered with 150,000 dead animals, we had over a million more to kill, and we were operating against a politically charged background, under the eye of the world's press, and initially totally without resources or direction.

My next overriding impression is of the individual worth of the men and women I was privileged to command, both military and civilian. I can think of only two people in the many I met in Cumbria whom I would in any way criticise. Without exception the remainder were desperate to win, either because they came from the community and their lives were inextricably interwoven with the tragedy or because they felt they were the professional representatives of the Army. It was merely necessary to obtain the facts, to analyse them clearly and to indicate the required courses of action in a clear and simple manner. Thereafter one needed only to stay on one's feet and continually override or bypass obstructions as they arose. In military terms, mission command works: if one explains what one wants doing and why, one can rely on one's subordinates to get it done one way or another and if they cannot they will come back having explored the other options in sufficient detail to allow one to revisit the plan immediately.

Finally I note to our cost, the penalties for failing to have a contingency plan for such operations. Perhaps it is time to revisit old procedures.

On a personal note, foot and mouth changed my life, seemingly irrevocably. I am frequently recognised, constantly approached for help and now work part time for the Rural Heritage Trust, a registered charity dedicated to regenerating the countryside by the provision of diverse and sustainable employment whilst maintaining the traditional backdrop for tourism. I wish it otherwise but my life, like that of so many others, is now interwoven with the disease.

Pauline Smith

Pauline Smith lives in Wiggonby near Wigton. The village is situated next to Great Orton Airfield which became a mass burial and slaughter site. This is her diary.

Saturday 24th March 2001

We heard on the news that MAFF was looking for an airfield to use to bury animals and for a pyre. Had a horrible feeling it would be Great Orton.

Sunday 25th March

We woke at about 7.30 a.m. to see army Land Rovers and cars going around the road to the airfield. We had our fears confirmed. It was to be Great Orton. By 10.00 a.m. many lorries with diggers and various earth moving machines arriving. By 11.00 a.m. men in white overalls are seen wandering around. Satellite dishes and TV vans start to arrive. Many cars seem to be arriving. Don't know what they are all up to. Police cars start to arrive and a lot of low-loaders with huge diggers and bulldozers are turning up. As we go to bed at 10.30 p.m. there are lights, reversing alarms and all sorts of things arriving in the dark.

Monday 26th March

We woke at 7.30 a.m. and have never seen so much activity around the

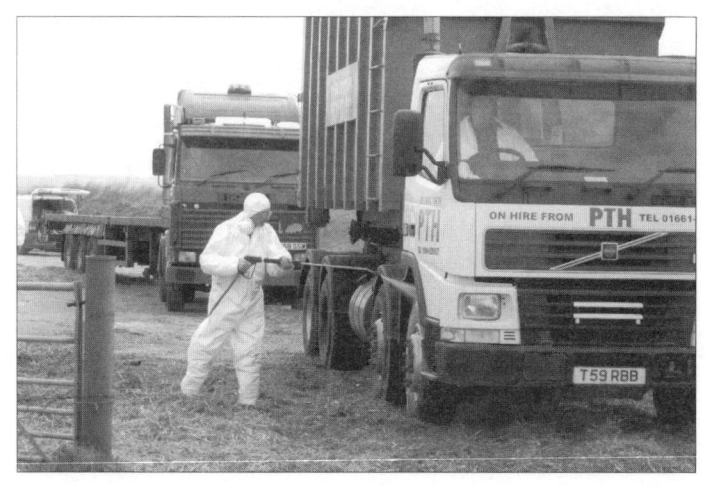

Photo: News & Star

Disinfecting became a way of life and a steady job for some people.

airfield. By the time the news was on TV they said 1200 dead sheep had been brought overnight. At least we didn't have to see that. 8.00 a.m. and many lorries with covered backs start to arrive. We have a horrible feeling they are the lorries with the dead animals in. The TV vans start to turn up. Some had been there late the night before, possibly all night. The graves they are working on at the minute are out of sight but no doubt they soon will be in sight. The TV crew says the smell is unbearable but we can't smell anything at home as the wind is in our favour.

All morning things are arriving; big bales, pens to put animals in, tankers of all description. There is a tanker at the entrance gate spraying the surrounding area. It's like a crowd control water cannon. The police have put up 'no waiting' signs around the entrance as the TV vans and cars were causing a roadblock. A big double arm hydraulic platform has arrived and a camera crew is now aloft overlooking the site. There are two or three helicopters in the sky and also a light aircraft. We have heard that Nick Brown is in Carlisle. He might be in one of the helicopters.

There is a rumour that the live sheep are being brought for slaughter tomorrow. We are going out for the day so I hope we won't see that but I suppose we will have to at some time. There are a lot of diggers and bulldozers on the runway waiting to start work. A lot of men in white overalls. It's like a set from a nuclear disaster movie. The sheep and lambs in the surrounding fields graze happily unaware of their fate, I hope. Reporters are going around looking for somebody to talk to them. Nobody, especially the farmers, feels much like talking.

Late afternoon, a lot of Portakabins and portable loos and a lorry load of dead sheep are in the queue to get into the site. Still more tankers arriving. Let's hope we never have to see this again. Life goes on as normal as possible.

Wednesday 28th March

It was too late on Monday to put in the diary, but a lot of concrete blocks arrived on the back of a lorry. I have no idea what they are for. I woke very early on Tuesday the 27th because we went out for the day; there were lots of lights, but it was too dark to see what was going on. We passed convoys of lorries on the M6 carrying dead animals. We got home at about 8.00 p.m. and it was too dark to see anything. A friend rang late on Tuesday evening and said a huge tent had been put up and could we see it from home? Luckily, we can't see it as that is where the slaughtering is going on.

Today we can see a pit being prepared; the diggers are scraping away the topsoil ready to dig the grave pit. Another huge lorry full of big bales has turned up. The TV camera crew are on the platform high in the sky waiting for the live sheep to arrive. They say only sheep are to be buried and cows are to be burnt on the pyres. A mobile cafe has set up shop by the press vans, no doubt making a bob or two out of them.

We have heard this morning that Hespin Wood is to be used for the burial of animals and also the forest near Lockerbie. I never realised how many dead animals there could be. At about 11.45 a.m. the lorries carrying the live sheep start to arrive. The camera crew is getting shots from every angle, even through the slots in the sides of the lorries. How sad. Since then it's been a steady stream of sheep arriving. Even small pick-ups towing small cattle trailers arrive. It looks like bring-your-own; it must be very upsetting for the farmers or whoever is bringing them.

At about 2.15 p.m. a lot of cars pull up. Cameramen and sound crews are very active as an army big-wig is to pay a visit - by the way, the police have put a ticket on all the cars! As I look up again, two more lorries full of sheep have just turned into the gate. I wish all of the press reports would be the same. Some say cattle are to come as well, but now it's only sheep. What next! I have not heard anything about pigs yet but I did hear on the news that some llamas have been slaughtered today because they were in a danger zone.

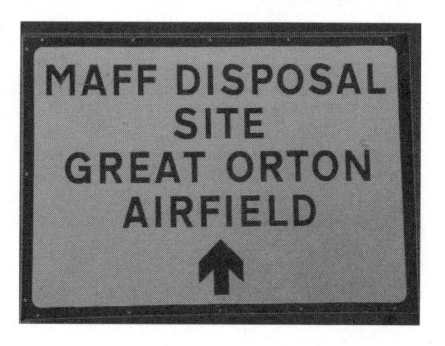

MAFF DISPOSAL SITE GREAT ORTON AIRFIELD ↑

Thursday 29th March

At 2.00 p.m. as I look out of the window there are eight 4-tier lorries loaded with sheep queuing to get into the site. The sheep must be terrified. In the same queue are three lorries full of dead animals. In a field just in front of the airfield a sheep has had a lamb, it lays very still and I secretly hope it's already dead because if not, it soon will be. A 4x4 is towing a small trailer with a few more live sheep. Another huge lorry, with a load of orange and white bollards is in the queue; they are being used to mark a route around the car parking area.

The whole site seems to be alive with bulldozers and diggers. A very large building has been put up by the tent. I am pleased we can't see the sheep in the pens waiting to be shot. Two more lorries full of sheep join the queue. There must be thousands arriving. Another light aircraft is in the sky doing a bit more filming, no doubt. A big tanker keeps coming and going carrying water. We know that because we passed him as he was topping up from a hydrant. The roads in the area are getting bad. They are not wide enough for two cars to pass, never mind the big lorries that come up here.

The farmer's Mum has just been to see the sheep in the front field. She seems to walk very slowly and sadly around the sheep, just to see if they get up and move. They do, but probably not for much longer. It must be heartbreaking. I am going to do some ironing now and have a last look at the sheep at the back of the house. It won't be much longer for them either.

A small mast has been erected in the parking area, no doubt to make communications a lot easier. Every time you look up there are more dead arriving. You can't help but keep looking, secretly hoping it's a bad dream and you'll wake up and all will be back to normal. When we go to bed the whole place is aglow with lights; it must be 24-hour slaughtering.

Friday 30th March

We woke at about 7.15 a.m. opened the curtains and the first thing we see is three wagons full of dead animals and by 7.30 another three 4-tier sheep wagons and three more wagons of dead. I don't know how many we have missed, but this is only the start of the day. How many more are there to come? We spoke to a girl last night whose Dad is doing some of the lorry driving; apparently he is earning £40 an hour. I don't think I could do it for a £100 an hour. But they have to earn it while they can because soon there will not be a lot of work for them.

The site's very busy this morning, more lorries with hardcore arriving. The camera crew are on the platform doing a live report on the news at the minute and about five minibuses have gone up for a shift change, probably more vets and slaughter men. It's nearly as busy as a major motorway. I am going shopping now at 11.00 a.m.

Back home and it's now 5.00 p.m. On my way home there was a strange car parked outside our neighbour's farm. It could be a visitor, but have got a horrible feeling it wasn't. Within half an hour the slaughter men were there. That's it, foot and mouth is now in the village. We feel very sad and sorry for them, but don't really want to believe it until we hear it confirmed on the news. We will speak to them in the morning, but I don't know how we will get the words out. You feel as if there has been a death in the family.

The dead are still arriving in convoy for the airfield, and in the queue are more live sheep. Thousands must have arrived today. The TV crews seem to have gone at the minute, probably up to Dumfries and Lockerbie where new pits are being dug. I never realised so much room would be needed.

Saturday 31st March

It's rainy and windy this morning. The weather suits the mood, miserable. It's 7.00 a.m. and the slaughterers' van is still at the farm. Apparently they were there until 10.30 p.m. last night. We sit in bed and have a coffee only to watch the convoy start again. At one stage there were ten lorries queuing. By the time we get downstairs and look out of the back windows we see the farmer's son stacking the dead cows in the field ready for a pyre later in the week. It's going to be at the bottom of the field where we can't see it. Thank God for that.

The telephone rings and as I stand talking they come out of the farm to round up and slaughter the few sheep and lambs they had in the front field. It was very sad seeing the lambs try to run away. They left them where they died, in a gateway. We went to Carlisle to get a few flowers and a bottle of whisky for the family. On the way to Carlisle we passed a field with a load of dead cows stacked up like black and white dominoes. When we got home, we met the farmer's wife at the farm gate. She looked very tired and pale and no doubt felt like it. We paid our respects,

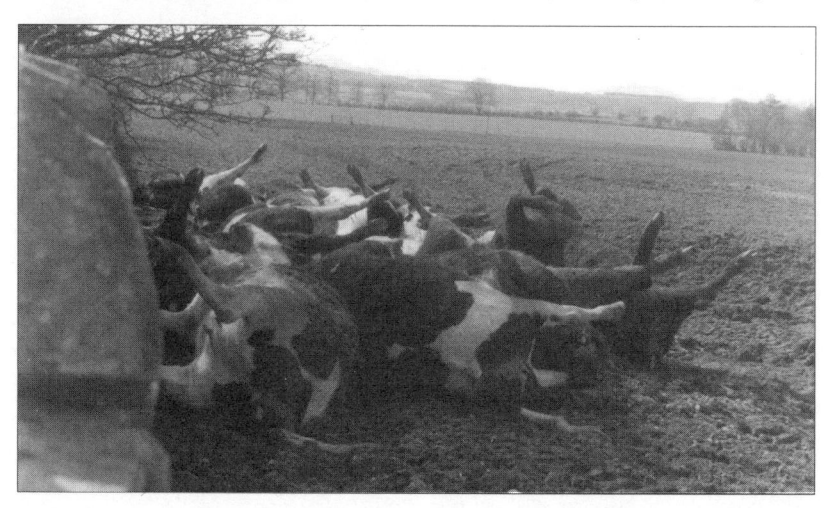

Photo: Nick Green

Piles of carcasses became all too common

had a chat mainly about F&M. We don't know what else to talk about at a time like this.

Sunday 1st April

April Fool's day and I was hoping it would be an April Fool's joke, but it's no joke. The cows are being stacked up ready for the pyre. It must be very sad to take them to the pyre yourself. They must be very strong. As I look up towards the killing field the TV crew are doing a live interview for 'Frost on Sunday' with the army Brigadier who is in charge. Only 9.30 a.m. and already the convoy of lorries full of sheep are arriving for slaughter. There are about 17 lorries lined up waiting to tip the dead. I don't know what the hold up is. Radio broadcasts have been appealing for more lorry drivers to help as there is a backlog of animals waiting to be buried. Some have been waiting two weeks; they must be in a terrible state by now. According to the news, they have already buried 50,000.

Monday 2nd April

Today we have found out why the loads have been building up; some of them contain young cows. They are waiting for the outcome of a meeting to see if they will allow burial whilst the older cows will still have to be burnt. On the news they are reporting 20 lorries queuing, but with our telescope we can see about 50. The TV vans are all coming back because they will want to be first with shots of the young cows being buried if the meeting allows this. The cab units of the lorries have all returned ready to hitch up and tip the loads; the outcome of the meeting must be for burial. We have also heard a traffic report on the local radio about road congestion in the Great Orton area. It is worse than Spaghetti Junction only with more death. The TV news never did show the young cows being buried. It must have been out of sight. Fifteen thousand dead animals are waiting to be picked up and God knows how many more are to be slaughtered.

Tuesday 3rd April

We have heard on the news that a load of animals buried in a field at Durham have got to be dug up as a watercourse has been polluted. Imagine the job the army has to do. I just hope they got the sums right when they decided to bury at Great Orton.

The farmer next door is still moving cattle to the bottom of the field where the pyre is located. I am so glad we won't have to see the animals on the pyre; the smoke will be bad enough. There are still a lot of live sheep arriving, but the lorries carrying the dead animals seem to be easing off. It's now down to one or two at a time, instead of five or six. A big lorry load of drainpipes arrive in the afternoon. What have they learnt from the Durham fiasco?

Wednesday 4th April

We sat in bed this morning watching the convoy of minibuses, cars and army Land Rovers arriving plus five loads of dead animals and it's still only 7.30 a.m. While we were having our breakfast a sheep transporter came and slowed down by our house and a horrible feeling came over us. We just knew they had come for our neighbour's sheep on the other side of our house, the ones I was watching while doing my ironing. There was a lot of noise while rounding them up. I kept telling myself it must be a better place where they are going. All that leaves is the forty sheep in the front field which I hope have another day left, but no doubt their days are numbered. The dead sheep have been moved this morning from the field gateway.

I am looking up towards the airfield and notice a large reel of plastic drainpipe has been delivered. I am sure something has come of the Durham fiasco. Out of the back of the house, we can see three plumes of smoke; it's a good job the wind is in our favour. More diggers are arriving at the airfield and on Radio Cumbria they are appealing for more lorry drivers and operators to work on the site. The job has turned out to be a massive earthworks and at the end of this there will be a lot of tired, stressed and traumatised people about.

Friday 6th April

Late last night we noticed bright lights at the bottom of the farmer's field and the pyre was lit late in the evening. I could not get to sleep thinking about the animals and the smoke. It was awful. Your imagination runs wild. I can't think how the farmer and his family feel.

Anyway, when we woke this morning, the first thing we did was check the wind and it was blowing the smoke away from us. Thank God for that. As we have our coffee in bed, we notice the usual convoy of cars and minibuses start to arrive and we listen to the TV news. This morning we are going to Carlisle and we will have to drive through the smoke of the pyre. It will be awful. On the way we meet a roadblock and have to turn around and find another route. They were killing animals at another farm on the way to Carlisle.

A couple of hours later when we got back home the wind had changed, blowing from the north. The smell was awful, not from the pyre but from the dead animals at the airfield. We unloaded the car very quickly and battened down the hatches. Thank goodness for good double-glazing. I don't know how the men can work in that smell all day.

I have not noticed so many wagons today but a lot of work is going on around the edge of the site. It looks like drainage being put in.

We have just had a call from a farmer up the road who has come down with F&M. We had sent him a card and paid our respects. He was ringing to say thanks and to tell us it had made his Mum so poorly with her heart trouble that she had to go to hospital. As if F&M was not bad enough. He is on the farm on his own and we told him if we could help in any way to let us know. He thanked us but said he had plenty of food in, as he had feared the worst. Now he is in quarantine, but not sure for how long.

It's a very dull and dismal day today and it's keeping the pyre smoke close to the ground, like a fog. We could do with some sunshine to make a bad job brighter.

Saturday 7th April

We woke this morning to a very wet day. The wind is from the north and the airfield is very muddy. The pyre at the back of the house is still smoking. The rain has done nothing. It just shows how hot it must be.

We have heard on a TV news report that a huge pyre is to be built at Longtown on the old airfield capable of burning thousands of carcasses a

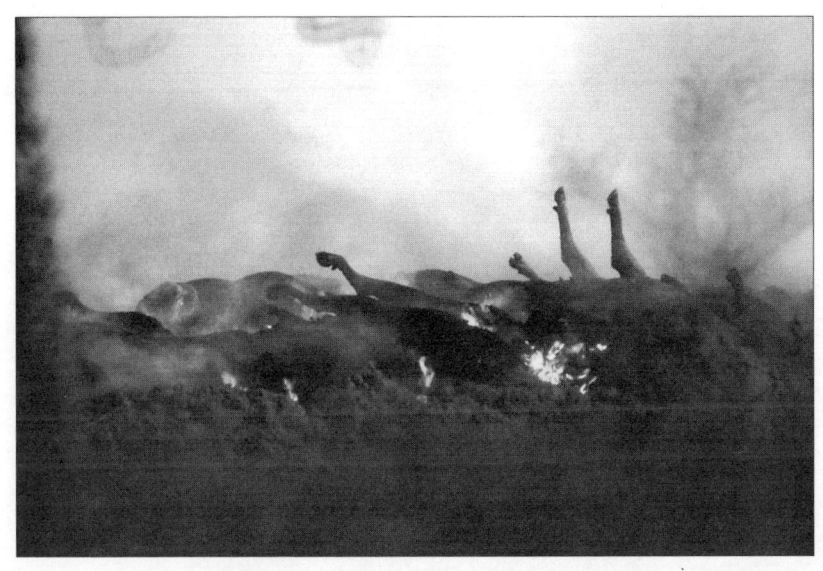

Photo: News & Star

day. The poor people of Longtown, haven't they suffered enough? Also on the news was an report about a farmer who lives down the road at the back of our house. He's blocked the road in protest due to the lorries continually passing his farm while he's had a yard full of dead decomposing cows for over a week. I think they were moved very shortly after this. Well done. I bet some of the TV crews are down there reporting on the incident. They love a bit of bother.

Monday 9th April
We are getting the smell this morning from the killing fields at Great Orton because the wind is in the north. We soon shut the windows and have our coffee in a stuffy room. About 10.30 a.m. the wind has changed to the south-east and now we can smell the remains of the pyre. It still smells of fleece and flesh and that is after burning for four days. Anyway, the sheep in the front are still with us, hopefully for another day or two.

Thursday 12th April
I wish I wasn't looking out of the window. A sheep wagon has just pulled up and, yes, it's the last day for the sheep opposite. They have done well to last as long as they have. I don't watch them being loaded but wish them a happier life wherever they are going. That is now Wiggonby empty of sheep. It's all so sad.

Friday 13th April
Good Friday. No way! It's a very Bad Friday. Our other farming neighbour has come down with F&M. The last cattle to go in Wiggonby. At about 9.00 a.m. six big lorries pull up on the road outside our house and they slaughter the animals. They are being taken straight away. In a way I am pleased because there won't be a pyre. I decide to go out and try to miss it, but I have a last look at the ladies, such fine cows, chewing their cud and grazing the silage heap. I wish I hadn't done that. I cried all the way to Carlisle. When I got back from shopping they had gone but there are four more wagons still waiting. You can hear the tractor, then the reversing alarm, then the thud as they land in the back of the wagon; it's such a sad end for such lovely animals. We are going to ring them tomorrow as I am sure today they won't want to talk to anybody. I look up the airfield and the usual convoy of wagons is arriving. Is there no end to it?

Wednesday 18th April
Well, Easter is over and there has not been much change. The minibuses, Land Rovers and cars arrive in convoy, sheep wagons are turning up and

it's still only 7.00 a.m. Last night we went round and had a brandy or two with the farmer and his wife. On the way there the smell was very strong from the airfield but on the way home, it was a little better - I think it may have been the brandy. The farmer's wife looks very sad and upset. I think he is too but he's trying to keep a brave face in front of people. I am sure they will get through it. Like many other farmers, they are a strong breed.

Anyway, the day goes on as normal. More drainpipes are being delivered; they will have a hell of a drainage system on site when it's all over!

Thursday 19th April

Late yesterday afternoon a large pyre was lit at Brocklebank near Wigton. It's so big at night it looks like a scene from the blitz, a fiery glow in the night sky. On the late TV news we learnt that there would be no more pyres in Cumbria. They lit that one because it had already been built. There have been health scares and until investigations have been carried out, no more pyres are to be lit. How must the people of Longtown feel after all the smoke that they have had to endure?

Sunday 22nd April

This morning seems very quiet. The cars and minibuses are arriving, but not much digger or bulldozer activity. You can see them just sitting on the runway. I have not seen any wagons carrying dead animals and only a couple of the live sheep wagons. It's definitely slowing down. I am sure they must have caught up with the backlog of dead. The whole site seems quiet, not many people moving about. It seems strange after all the activity.

Tuesday 24th April

Late last night I looked out of the front windows and even the lights were dimmer than usual. There were no flashing lights or any movement like other nights. It's very strange. This morning two large tankers with 'Effluent Services Ltd.' on one side and 'Working to Protect the Environment' on the other side arrived and I wonder if they are pumping the liquid from the pits and if so, where is it going? Four covered wagons have just stopped on the road outside at the farm next door. It must have been a horrible moment to relive for the farmer. They must have lost their way.

Three buzzards are circling around in the sky like vultures in a western film, waiting to come down to the carcasses. I wish it was a western being made because at the end of the day everybody and everything could get up and go home.

Thursday 26th April

I had a coffee in Tesco's cafe in Carlisle today. It was like being in the NAAFI, so many tables were occupied by soldiers having a cup of tea. I have never seen so much army activity around Carlisle.

Today Mr Blair paid a visit to Rosehill to speak to the chosen few, not the people that matter, the farmers. They have done a U-turn today on the culling program and now it's only going to be sheep on contiguous farms and not the cattle. A farmer talking on Radio Cumbria was gutted; his animals went yesterday and as he said 'they must have known about the change in policy'. He was heartbroken and like myself listening to him, many people must have been touched by what he said. Talk about vote grabbing. It seems to me the decision was made after pictures of a twelve-day-old calf were shown on TV. It had survived the cull of its mother and the rest of the herd. They want to save it from death. It's a lovely calf but so were the thousands that have already been lost.

Friday 27th April

This is the last day that I am writing this diary as today is the last day for Brigadier Birtwistle. He is retiring. He has done a good job in getting everything organised and getting it all to run smoothly. Therefore, I will finish with my thoughts.

They have killed off many thousands of sheep, cattle, pigs and rare breeds too, but that hardy rare breed the Cumbrian farmer will never be killed off. They will survive and come back. Even at this minute it must seem impossible for some, but time is a great healer. We will never forget, but you will survive. I have nothing to do with farming but I have felt very involved.

NO ENTRY: Animal Disease Control Precautions

Margaret Redmond & Jacqui Spanton

Margaret Redmond and Jacqui Spanton wrote this poem after meeting regularly at St James' Church, Ireby. The church became an important focal point for the community and each day at the height of the crisis a retired minister led prayers for those affected by foot and mouth. At one time villagers were praying for a list of more than fifty families from the Uldale, Ireby and Boltongate area.

The Uldale Lament

Do you ken Peel's Cumberland
With its wide green fells?
Do you ken Peel's hame
With its becks and gills?
Do you ken this land
Where sorrow wells?
Oh! They're building the fires
For the burning pyres
In Cumbria.

Do you ken the farmsteads
Of stone so grey?
Do you ken the shepherds
With their flocks a sway?
There's nothing there now
They've all been taken away.
Oh! They're lighting the fires
For the burning pyres
In Cumbria.

They took our sheep and lambs
So the cattle could stay,
Then they slaughtered a thousand cattle
All in a day,
And strong men weep at shattered dreams
While trees break leaf by crystal streams.
Oh! Empty fields and empty byres
Gone to feed the burning pyres
Of Cumbria.

Do you ken Peel's Cumberland
As it was yesterday?
Do you ken Peel's hame
Before MAFF and others came?
There's nothing there now
All taken away.
Oh! Empty hearts and empty byres
Because of the burning pyres
Of Cumbria.

Do you ken the lambs as they jump in the air?
Joy in their hearts without a care.
Do you ken the yows in the sunset's glare
To be met with the sorrow in the morning.

Do you ken wintered cows coming in, rush and push?
They look to their fields of green grass lush.
Do you ken their eyes full of gentle trust
To be met with the sorrow in the morning.

Do you ken the love flowing through our land
From friends who care and God's faithful hand?
Do you ken new beasts blaring, isn't this grand?
For there will be joy in the morning.

Dr Jim Cox

Dr Jim Cox is a GP in Caldbeck.

When foot and mouth disease was first diagnosed at Heddon on the Wall, I was relieved that the outbreak was well away from home. Driving to Newcastle soon afterwards, I drove past the funeral pyre and through the cloud of smoke that engulfed the A69. The scene was distressing and I stopped to take a photograph, little suspecting that the sight and smell of burning carcases would rapidly become commonplace.

Within days the disease was recognised in Cumbria and it was not long until it was diagnosed in animals in Raughton, the first case in a farm in our practice. Within a few weeks we had well over 100 farms with confirmed cases - at one stage one in seven of all the cases in the UK. Like most people, I was unprepared, shocked and upset in a way that I had not experienced before. I am used to dealing with accidents, tragedy, death and grief - but never before on this scale. My colleagues in the practice were equally affected, yet most of us were only experiencing the tragedy secondhand. We were better off than most people.

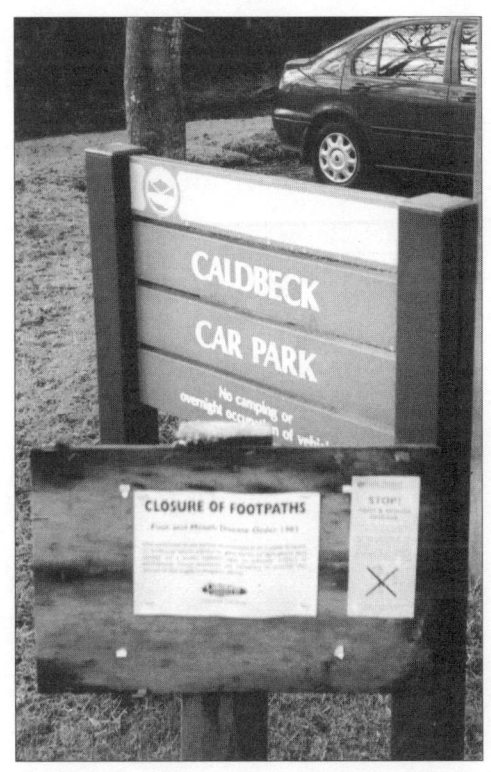

For a while, fewer people came to the surgery as people restricted their movements to essential journeys only. But every consultation took twice as long because it was invariably necessary to discuss the foot and mouth epidemic as a lengthy preliminary. My partners, our nurses, receptionists and everyone at the surgery spent hours listening to people's stories, in person and on the phone. We thought that it was important that we did so. Several members of the practice 'team' live on farms and were personally affected by the culling of their animals and some were unable to come to work for a time.

It soon became obvious that foot and mouth disease impacted on almost everyone. Many farmers had confirmed disease on their farms. Many more were 'taken out' in MAFF's slow and inadequate attempts to control the epidemic. Others were struggling to protect their animals from infection by isolating themselves from the rest of the world, and some still are. Whole families were in distress and some were split up as children were 'evacuated' as in wartime, in attempts to allow them to continue their education and take exams. Foot and mouth disease seemed to be the only topic of conversation.

As an initial response to the epidemic, we phoned each farm with confirmed disease to offer sympathy and support. However, animals were being culled on many more farms than had the disease and there was no way of identifying them. Only those farms with confirmed disease were listed on the MAFF website. And, of course, not only farmers were feeling the strain. Everybody was affected. As an illustration, an extremely stoical, retired woman cried as I told her the bad news that a long dormant cancer had spread and was inoperable. I was only partly surprised when she explained that she was not crying for herself or her future, but she was crying because she was devastated by the effect the foot and mouth epidemic was having on animals and people.

The practicalities of providing health care changed. If we set foot on an infected farm we were 'dirty' doctors or nurses and not allowed to visit uninfected farms for the next seven days. MAFF quickly reduced this to five then to three days, although they never explained the logic. I treated a woman for severe migraine with headache and vomiting in a car by their farm gate at midnight. She simply wanted relief from her symptoms and refused examination. Neither she nor her husband wanted visitors on their uninfected farm. Sadly they 'went down' only days later. At another farm gate I treated a slaughter man who had dislocated his shoulder killing sheep. We learned that children had developed new games that reflected their new lives, for example playing 'sheep' which mainly involved getting shot.

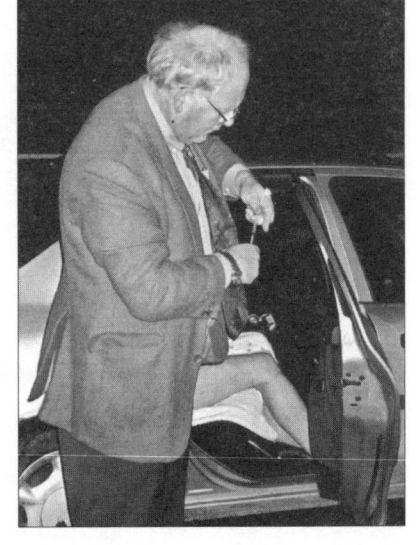

At a practice meeting we discussed what we could do to help. By phoning farmers whose names had come up on the Internet as confirmed cases, we were only reaching a minority. Not only were we failing to contact all the other farmers whose stock had been slaughtered, but also we usually contacted only one of several family members who were affected. Furthermore, we had not made contact with all the non-farmers, including those whose livelihood had been devastated by the slump in tourism.

We also realised that, for many people, a trip to the surgery was a rare opportunity to escape their MAFF-enforced or self-enforced exile and meet other people.

We decided to write to every household in the practice to offer assistance if required and to provide contact numbers for 'help-lines' etc. We also laid on tea and coffee in the surgery waiting room and encouraged everyone, particularly the most isolated people, to use the opportunity of a visit to the surgery to stay and chat with others. There was no shortage of conversation!

There have been no new cases in our practice area for many weeks. Some older farmers without family to follow them will retire. Others are still disinfecting their farms. A significant number of farms remain uninfected, although most have lost their sheep. Their predicament is probably the hardest at the moment.

The tourist trade in the northern Lake District is precarious and although many Lake District footpaths are open again, the northern fells remain overgrown and out-of-bounds. The epidemic has highlighted the relationships between, and crucial interdependence of agriculture, stewardship of the countryside and tourism.

There is a lot of discussion going on, from around the farmhouse table to Downing Street. But still no one knows what the future will be. I passionately hope that there will be a place for local young people who can, like the lamented 'hefted' or 'heafed' sheep, stay put and continue to farm and nurture the countryside and preserve its traditions and culture. But the future will undoubtedly be different.

If one were to believe the national press, one would think that the crisis was over, but it is not. The infection does not appear to be under control.

Depression and gloom are commonplace in the best of winters. I fear a hard winter ahead. This year (2001 - 2002) many people will be without their animals, their regular work or an income. I only hope that if they are desperate, they will seek professional help and not, as stoical Cumbrians tend to do, struggle silently and sometimes fatally. We are still near the beginning of a long journey towards a different future.

Heidi Jackson

Heidi Jackson's parents, Nan and Arnold Savage, are hill farmers at Whelpo which lies between Caldbeck and Uldale. After a difficult decision in April they gave up their sheep to the voluntary cull. Heidi helped them gather the flock in and sent this email to close friends later that same day.

----- Original Message -----
From: Heidi & David Jackson
Sent: Saturday, April 07, 2001 11:31 PM
Subject: F & M Update - Dreadful Day

Friends

F & M Update

Yesterday was the day we had all been dreading. The wagons were coming to take the healthy sheep to be slaughtered. Beatrix and I stayed over at Caldbeck. Mam looked after Beatrix in the morning whilst I helped Dad gather the sheep and lambs up to be loaded onto the wagons.

The whole process was so sad and terrible. Normally moving sheep and lambs at this time of the year is satisfying. Not yesterday - it was awful. I constantly had to fight back the tears. How Dad managed to cope I'll never know.

I was trying to take photos before it was all gone forever - all Dad & Mams hard work over the last 34 years. And the hard worked showed - the sheep have never looked so well, fit, healthy and prime examples - something that can only come from the work of a lifetime.

4 wagons turned up, 3 huge ones and a smaller one, for the lambs. That was one of the things that was upsetting me the most, the fact that the sheep and lambs were going to be separated before they were taken from the farms. All I could think about was how stressed they would be because of this, and the noise. The sheep shouting for the lambs, the lambs shouting for their mothers.

We got the sheep loaded, 680 or so. But when I walked into the shed whilst the little wagon backed up to the shed door I finally broke down. The sight of hundreds of lambs all together shouting for their mothers was just too much. One of the worst things was the twin lambs from a sheep that was giving birth as the sheep had been rounded up just minutes earlier. The sheep would have been a good mother as it was really reluctant to leave them and difficult to load. The poor little lambs didn't even get a chance to suckle.

Everything was finally loaded and driven off - a sad, sad morning. One that I'll never forget. A morning that unfortunately so many other people are also having to go through at the moment up here. Any time you see a wagon of sheep up here you know it's their last trip - they are the only live animals allowed to be moved, the sad thing is you see them all the time so many are being culled.

The only thing worse for a farmer than sending his entire healthy flock for slaughter must be to see his flock come down with foot and mouth and have them shot in front of him and then to be piled up in his farmyard waiting to be burnt or buried. Every time I get upset I have to try to remember this. What we did was to try to stop this.

The way the disease is spreading relentlessly makes you think that it is inevitable that you will get it. Another case was confirmed in Caldbeck yesterday - right in the centre of the village. When will it stop?

Part of me feels guilty for writing this to you all, David is in Australia at the moment and it's hard to talk to him and I need to share this with people I care about.
The other part of me wants people to have an idea of what it is really like for people affected by this.

I hope you don't mind.

Thanks for listening.

Heidi.

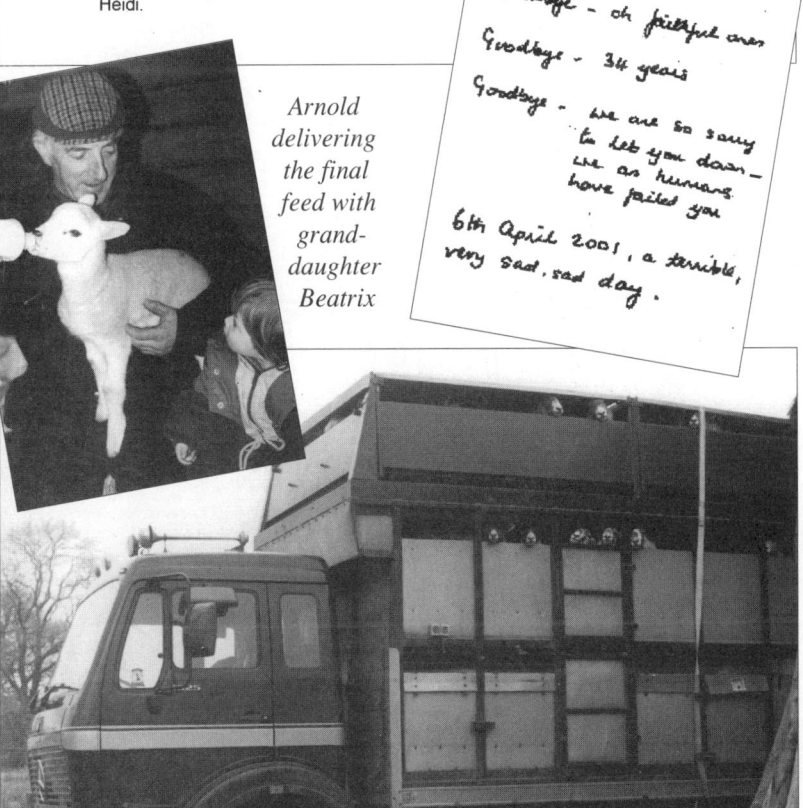

Arnold delivering the final feed with granddaughter Beatrix

Goodbye - oh faithful ones
Goodbye - 34 years
Goodbye - we are so sorry to let you down - we as humans have failed you.
6th April 2001, a terrible, very sad, sad day.

Debbie Steele

Debbie Steele was coordinator of the Cumbria Stress Information Network which ran a 24 hour phone help-line during the foot and mouth outbreak. They received thousands of calls from people who had nowhere else to turn.

How can you start to write about the impact of foot and mouth disease? When I first heard that the virus had been reported it seemed like it might be something that would be horrible for those affected, but that would surely only affect an isolated few, and would be brought under control in no time at all. Wouldn't it? But the disease quickly spread with little or no time for formal plans. At Cumbria Stress Information Network we were too busy trying to change the way we worked to meet the needs of the situation to allow time for panic. It quite literally changed overnight. I was asked to go onto BBC Radio Cumbria on the 6th March to say what we could offer to those worried about the possible effects of foot and mouth on their lives and livelihoods. 7.00 a.m. is not a good time for me... and when asked if we were going to extend the hours of the phone line, it was automatic to respond positively. So we went from maybe 2 calls a month from the public to up to 50 a day. These came at all times of the day or night, and could not always simply be passed on to somebody else to handle.

One of the things that impressed me most was the dignity of those who called. Many had just been told that they had lost their livelihoods and potentially a way of life that had been evolved over generations, and yet here they came quietly asking for information and advice.

Frequently there was barely time to log details of one call before the next came through. Often those calling offered help and support to others so that they might not suffer in the same way as they had themselves.

The calls were extremely moving and these are just a few examples that represent those we got every day of the week:-

The farmer who asked simply for somebody to talk with him while his cattle were slaughtered outside. We spoke for three and a half hours and at the end of the call he quietly said that it was time for him to get on. He called again a few days later to thank me for my time. It was that second call that brought me to tears. How could somebody who had lost so much still find time to thank somebody who had so little that they could really give?

The quiet dignity of the man who thought his business, so reliant on tourism, was going to fail taking with it his family's life savings.

The call from a lady asking for help feeding her cattle. When this was resolved we asked if she was managing for shopping. It was only then that she revealed that she and her father had lived on bread and butter for a week as she had nothing else to feed them on and no money to buy it with anyway. Her first consideration had been for her animals.

The mother who rang to ask for support for her daughter who was quarantined on a farm with young children. We knew about the daughter already. She had rung earlier that day to ask that somebody try to make contact with her mother who would be feeling lonely and isolated without her family to visit her.

Every call gave a different perspective on the full horror of foot and mouth.

We received countless offers of help and through these people we formed a small group of volunteers who helped to staff the phones 24 hours a day. It should be borne in mind that these people had often been deeply affected by the disease themselves, and yet selflessly gave of their time and efforts.

It is impossible to thank all those whose kindness to others and to myself at this time was so important, but without the support of everybody from Voluntary Action Cumbria, my partner Ian, and the volunteers who were always ready with a listening ear, or a shoulder to cry on, I do not think I could have continued. Thank you is inadequate at this time.

By the end of August we had received in excess of 2,700 calls, each one of those from a real person like you or me, an individual trying to cope with a disease that wrought havoc amongst those it touched.

My most lasting memories of this disease will be the care and compassion shown to others suffering by those who are often affected even more. The way that families and communities have pulled together to fight the disease and its effects for so long and so hard, taking each day and its accompanying problems as they came.

We still have a way to go and I for one am still learning new things daily.

NO ENTRY: Animal Disease Control Precautions

BBC ONLINE
Text only

foot & mouth

THURSDAY
19th October 2000

A-Z Index | Search

Main Sites ▼

BBC Homepage
England
▸ **Radio Cumbria**
Sport
Station Tour
Foot and Mouth
Gardening
About Radio Cumbria
Presenter Profiles
Daily Schedule
Photo Album
The Poser
Webcam
Weather
Look North

my BBC

Feedback

Help

Like this page?
Send it to a friend!

Marie Stockdale

Marie is a farmer near Sandale, west of Wigton. How has the crisis changed her life?

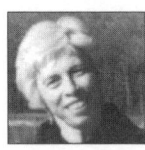

Marie Stockdale comes from a Cumbrian farming family. She and Alan Barrow live at Pow Heads, on the fells overlooking the Solway Firth, with their sons Fred, 11, and Eric, 6. They have diversified, in the last 2 years, from traditional farming to directly retailing home-produced meat and poultry through a farm shop and farmers' markets.

Quick Links:
April: Mon 2nd Weds 4th Fri 6th Sun 8th Fri 13th Easter Day Easter Monday Tues 24th
May: Mon 14th
August: Fri 31st

Monday 2nd April

This is nearly too late to start a Foot and Mouth diary but I can tell you about the Foot and Mouth Fandango, if you like. When we looked on the MAFF website this afternoon we realised it is now closing in on us on three sides.
This farm sits on top of a hill and there is a case now at the bottom of our hill.

It seems vaccinaton, if it comes, will come to late for us. Bowing to the inevitable, we made the decision, unbelievable 2 weeks ago, that now we should go for a voluntary cull. Culling us won't protect many people now that it has reached Caldbeck Common, but we do have pigs and they supposedly create "plumes" of infection, which can't be a good thing for the neighbourhood if we get it.

We also don't like the stories we hear locally of infected animals destroyed but left in their byres or wherever they happened to be for nearly 2 weeks. We have young children and that is a trauma and health risk we would like to avoid, at least culled animals are moved off the farm

So, feeling very emotional, I set about the practicalities: knowing it is impossible to get through to MAFF in Carlisle I rang the Foot and Mouth Hotline, they gave me a number in Newcastle which proved impossible to get through to. Dead end. Speaking to our vet about something totally unconnected, I mentioned this fact and he said,
"Oh, that's the wrong number, that's the Welfare Cull number, you want to phone the local auction mart."
Easy enough.

They said they thought only sheep were being dealt with in the voluntary cull, phone the head of the voluntary

BBC Radio Cumbria

▸ YOUR WEATHER

Carlisle Five Day Forecast

▸ NEWS
Army seals Pakistani parliament
Political foes unite on Europe
Tanzania's Nyerere dies

▸ SPORT
Jenkins on course for world record
Kiwis survive for draw

▸ CONTACT DETAILS
Frequency:
95.6, 96.1 and 104.1 FM

BBC Radio Cumbria,
Annetwell Street,
Carlisle,
Cumbria.
CA3 8BB

Tel: 01228-592444
Phone-In: 01228-592592

and

Hartington Street,
Barrow-in-Furness,
Cumbria.
LA14 5JL

Tel: 01229-836767
Phone-In: 01228 592592

Editor: Nigel Dyson

Email:
radio.cumbria@bbc.co.uk

ABOUT ENGLISH REGIONS
Find out more about English Local Radio and Regional TV.

ACCOUNTABILITY
The BBC wants to hear from you

Cull to ask about pigs. He said I would need to talk to MAFF in Carlisle........who I know I won't be able to get through to. I think there's a hole in my bucket, dear Liza, a hole. I was no longer emotional, just tired and bewildered.

Now back to the normal world. There's a pet lamb to feed and I am a rather inadequate surrogate mother at the moment, a bit distracted. We both need a bit of luck.

Wednesday 4th April
It definitely feels like Them and Us. From our side the plan is not obvious. Today we had a phone call to say a Ministry Vet was on his way to check our animals.
Even at normal times this is an event that brings feelings of trepidation (it is amazing how any animal on the farm feeling slightly off-colour makes the effort to stagger forward to meet the illustrious visitor) so today we were really apprehensive. But nothing is the same any more. The vet arrives driving sporty little coupe and turns out to be a charming Italian. He wasn't very chatty at first but I expect he's a bit fed up of nervous farmers making jokes ("You know how the legionaries felt now,eh?...Hadrian's Wall, you know, ha,ha").

He had a good look round and all cattle, pigs, and sheep were given a clean bill of health even though one of last year's pet lambs trotted over with froth round it's mouth! Goodness knows what it had been up to but it must have been a bit surprised at the reaction it got: grabbed, turned on its back and 3 people trying to look into its mouth. It may decide to skip the pleasantries next time I go into the shed.

Thank goodness he didn't want to do that with any of the pigs. Our pigs are not in a pig shed, just in a barn, and some of them should have gone to the abattoir a month ago and are now getting very large. Without proper handling facilities we would have needed reinforcements to check any mouths.

All that remained was the form filling. To our surprise the form we were given turned out to be "Form D" which restricts movement of anything off the farm without a license. I only realised after he'd gone that we hadn't asked why we had got it! Not that it really matters, but we don't actually know which case has put us into a restricted area.

The upshot is that I have to try and speak to MAFF again to get a license to deliver the oven-ready poultry we were going to sell at Easter. I am filled with foreboding. I know people with large poultry sites are getting licenses easily enough but they are big business. To my amazement I get through to MAFF almost immediately. I think that's because we are now diverted to a Call Centre, the girl who answered gave me what I sincerely hope was incorrect advice and told me I would be called back. If she is correct we are going to have to eat our way through 50 turkeys, 200 chickens, and 100 ducks, of course we might be trampled to death by giant pigs before that.

Friday 6th April
I was printing the "Foot and Mouth – Keep Out" notice while Alan talked to his brother about the cull that is definitely going to happen shortly on his farm. When he put the phone down he held his hand out and said "Look at that!" It was shaking. It soon stopped but every now and then the enormity of it all comes home and the stress shows one way or another. I toyed with the idea of trying to find out what they are going to do about us but I have already been told twice by MAFF that I would be rung back about the poultry situation so it seems pointless to burden an obviously overloaded system with yet another enquiry when we will no doubt find out soon enough.

Went out for lunch and shopping instead. I've done more shopping and socialising in the last 2 months than I have in the last 2 years, I think. The military presence is very obvious, considering the numbers I have seen quoted (189 in this region). I suppose it is because they are concentrated in such a small area. It is surprisingly comforting. Brigadier Alex Birtwhistle is becoming a bit of a hero round here, probably because at last there is human being, with a name and a face and everything, who is organising things and things are happening.

For instance.... Janette in the village has been looking after some sheep for her sister because they are near Wigton, in an infected area, and were due to be culled, so contact with the farm had to be avoided. Even though they had been valued they could get no information from MAFF about when it was likely to happen. Janette was getting worried, feeding them was one thing but they were due to lamb any day. When the first one lambed she got a bit desperate. Exasperated, she wrote to "Brigadier Birtwhistle, The Old Airfield, Great Orton".

The following day she was phoned by an Engineer. Action. A bit shambolic,true - a trailer that could take 40 sheep arrived so, as there were 110, the whole operation took some time, in fact she was there for 7 hours. But there is a war on, you know. Not only that but the Italian vet told us that there are vets arriving from Canada and the USA so, finally, the Yanks are coming, just like old times! Let's hope they remembered to pack the chocolate and nylons and we can jitterbug the nights away.

Evening: Now we have heard that another, even closer, neighbour has it. A few weeks ago when you heard rumours they used turn out to be wrong, now they are almost always true. We have also heard that the valuer is coming tomorrow which means the sheep and pigs are going to be culled. As well as our regular "pink" pigs, we have a few Saddlebacks and I happened to see a pot Saddleback in the Upfront Gallery today (delicious lunch, interesting exhibition and open as normal), it was quite expensive but I'm glad I bought it.
Top of Page

Sunday 8th April
Well, it's arrived at the doorstep. The neighbour who has it has sheep in a field next to ours, just separated by a wire fence. I think all their animals are dead already. It was terrible to hear the blaring and bleating as they were all rounded up, knowing that it wasn't the usual quick trim or pedicure they were going in for.

I've been rung back about the poultry but I told the very helpful lady from Movement Licenses that I shouldn't waste her time because if we get the disease before the cull everything will have to go on the pyre anyway so the sensible thing seems to be to wait.

We should have been valued today for the so-called voluntary cull but when I told the valuer how the situation had developed, he said he would have to check because we might need a "dirty" valuer now and he was a "clean" one. Funny that, because when you think you've got it (which we do about ten times a day) it does feel "dirty".

Gates seem to have acquired an awful significance now. A red and white warning notice is pinned to each one along roads in infected areas. They are also used, with hurdles, to make the temporary pens for the slaughtermen to use and, when the hurdles are removed, a small group of carcases remains by the gate for a while. Quite shocking to see, especially when it is the sheep who have been part of your personal landscape for a long time. Finally, and I think it might become one of the images that will remain of this year, the unusual sight of gate after gate left open………. until who knows when!
Top of Page

Friday 13th April
I have been in charge of the lambing shed for the last 2 days while Alan pursues our other diversification: pressure washing on other farms. For 2 weeks he has been saying "what a great lambing, big fine twins", of course when I take over we hit a run of singles and if you have big twins, you get bigger singles. These often fail to adopt the recommended "nose between toes" diving position for birth and the head alone makes an appearance while the shoulders lodge. When this happens the anatomy of a sheep allows it to go about it's business as normal without any of the discomfort that I, for instance, would experience in similar circumstances, in fact it can show a turn of speed and an agility over hurdles that Sally Gunnell would envy. I am not what you would call match fit and I have had 4 of these reluctant mothers to lamb in 24 hours. When I caught the first one we both had to lie quietly for some minutes just to make sure neither of us was going to drop dead from a heart attack. The lamb then has to be pushed back where it came from (a procedure that makes both our eyes water) and realigned with head and fore feet coming together. Amazingly, the lamb is usually alive when it re-emerges.

Up until then I managed to avoid going in with the sheep much, I suppose I didn't want to get involved when they are all supposed to be going any day. The livestock has all been valued so it is just a question of time. In many ways it is not so hard for us because most of our stock is terminal and many would, in normal circumstances, have already have been sold through the farm shop We are not sentimental about sending our animals to the abattoir when they they reach maturity and peak condition but the mass slaughter of young, some very young, animals seems very unnatural and it feels as if we are going to fail in our duty to them. To be realistic, though, it may not be that different from the animals' point of view.

It was reassuring to read in the local evening paper, The News and Star, a slaughterman's description of the killing techniques used on farms. George, the slaughterman in question, works at our local abattoir so it was quite a shock to see him on the front page with the headline "The Man Who Must Silence The Lambs". He was pretty appalled by the headline, too,as he'd talked to the paper to put the record straight after reading sensationalised reports in the national press. When you go about your job in a professional and humane manner it must be very annoying being linked by suggestion with Hannibal Lecter. It sounds like it is very tense work, arriving on farms and not knowing what the handling facilities are going to be like, or the people - vets and farmers. But George and his team obviously feel a sense of responsibility to both farmer and livestock and have been managing to keep the stress on the animals to a minimum. We still don't know what is going to happen to our animals or when.

Sensational reporting is not limited to Britain, my sister tells me the main national newspaper in Italy had, on the front page, a photo of the "Road Closed" sign on the Thursby by-pass (for non-locals, we are talking here of a very small minor road) with the headline: "Great Orton Airport Closed". True enough I suppose, though, as it is a disused airfield, I shouldn't think anything larger than a microlight has landed on the since the war! Her friends in Italy seem to be under the impression that all our meat is infected and the country has gone vegetarian. I suppose to people who are not involved in agriculture in any way it is inevitable that Foot and Mouth is lumped with BSE as another health risk that Britain has inflicted on the world. A friend in Canada tells me that he gathers "military style travel restrictions are in force in the UK." ……….. Tony Blair has got his work cut out if he wants to present this country as the place, of all the places in the World, that YOU should choose for your holidays this year, when the newspapers have decided we are under siege. Which reminds me, where IS Kate Adie?
Top of Page

Easter Day
The sheep are going today. We trudged up the track to get them in. Alan kept quietly singing "It's the Final Countdown!" I wish he knew more than the first line. I think I caught a few bars of "The Last Train to Clarkesville" as well which shows the way his mind is working. The roundup went very well, sometimes ewes and lambs can be hellish to move.
The haulage company rang to discuss numbers and access. We were told "between 1 and 4pm". The first wagon arrived at 10.30am. He had no idea how many sheep there would be. To keep up the war analogy (and I don't seem to be able to avoid it) this must be Dunkirk…….owners of wagons, large and small, are being sent into the hills with orders to bring back sheep. As we look from our gate, to Ireby and beyond to the hills on the other side of the valley, there is hardly a sheep to be seen. It is an incredible operation being performed at high speed because Ireby is now the Front Line. The village is affected because the Ritson family have found infection in their sheep which means their herd of Dairy Shorthorns, now very rare, will be lost, along with 150 years of breeding. The cattle were not infected so

perhaps some semen can be saved. The other farm in the heart of the village, Willy and Anne Young's, who supply most of us with our milk, have been devastated to hear that their cattle are to go as "dangerous contacts." These make our losses seem fairly insignificant.

Our sheep get loaded, 300 sheep and 150 lambs, and my dislike of three-tier wagons is reinforced. They just don't want to go up on that top deck.

It is Easter Sunday. My mother said "Fancy taking them on Easter Sunday!" She then suggests I should tell Fred they are going to be resurrected as vultures and come back and eat us for doing this! I'm going to have to stop her watching "Buffy the Vampire Slayer", I fear for her mind.

A ministry vet rings to talk about slaughtering the pigs on the farm tomorrow (no facilities for taking live pigs to be culled) on the whole it is probably better for them to die here. We are very apprehensive, though.

Top of Page

Easter Monday

Alan walked round imaginary sheep this morning. I suggested he counts stonechats and wheatears. I also suggested that we need not worry about controlling the carrion crows now that we don't have any lambs.
My father had a soft spot for crows and he used to have some very tame ones coming to the garden, which I liked.
I knew what the answer was going to be, though, and, sure enough, if we are going to farm wildlife, we are going to have more and better birds than anyone else so we must keep the predators in check.
You can't keep a good peasant down.
It would be nice if we could get some curlews back, we will see if it is the silage-making that has driven them away if they reappear when we don't make any!

The invasion started with the Ministry Vet, then the MAFF official, then the slaughter team, then, finally, Cpl James Thompson, 22nd Regiment Royal Artillery Workshops, who will oversee the evacuation. It appears the main weapon in this theatre of operations is the mobile phone.

Chris, the vet, takes the opportunity to show us some pretty revolting pictures of diseased animals and tries to get through to us the difference between an "A" notice and the "D" notice we've become used to: it turns out we will have "A" on the pig shed, which means it will have to be cleaned out as an infected premises and "D" on the rest of the farm. He and Alan go off to turn the shed into a slaughterhouse and Kirwyn, the MAFF official, explains the clean-out to me. As Alan is a professional pressure washer the cleaning will not be a problem but this farm has been carefully sited between 2 small becks (or streams, as they would be known elsewhere). You can see that 200 hundred years ago this was a pretty smart move: fresh water into troughs and dirty water draining away, although nothing at Pow Heads ever works quite that efficiently. When Alan's mother arrived here the clean water was a trickle from a back kitchen tap and, when it rained, dirty water from the yard ran in at the back door and out at the front! The run off from washing the pig shed will obviously be unacceptable, Kirwyn thinks a lagoon may be necessary. I immediately picture palm trees, blue seas, sandy beaches, but, no, it seems a lagoon can also be a pond filled with a potent blend of slurry and disinfectant, not too many people queuing up to be Castaways here, I suspect. I cannot imagine how we will do it, but we will be given advice – something MAFF has plenty of and freely shares.

The slaughter team arrive and very soon we have no pigs, no sheep, just 16 cattle! As most of the cattle will be over thirty months when this is all over, they will be incinerated. We think they should go now. The vet thinks they should go now and predicts we will all meet again before long. The slaughtermen think they should slaughter them "seeing we're here". Common sense is not in charge, however, and the system is so overstretched cattle are only being taken out on the Front Line. Apparently the prediction is that, of the farms left behind with livestock, 80% will get Foot and Mouth. A new word for our vocabulary: "sentinel" – the cattle left behind will act as sentinels and show whether the disease is still present.

Alan lives in constant dread that someone will die of thirst on the premises, so there is an interlude while everyone is rehydrated with beer or coffee. The vet is forced to eat home-cured gammon, those James Herriot books have a lot to answer for! Finally we are left alone with our dead pigs and Alan has the sad task of dragging them out of the shed. As usual, Eric (6) wants to help his Dad. We do have a butchery so our children are used to seeing dead animals. Eric is given the job of carrying out the little piglets but, I tell him, they must be treated with respect even though they aren't alive. His reaction is to lay them out with their mother as if they were suckling. I know it will seem macabre to some and a fond mother may be a bit biased, but I thought that was rather touching.

Top of Page

Tuesday 24th April

Well, we're feeling a bit shell-shocked today. We've been "*Dorised*".
At 7 o'clock in the morning I was explaining our strange situation on Radio Cumbria, being left with 16 cattle, most of which would have to be incinerated when the Foot and Mouth outbreak is over because they will be over 30 months old (BSE regulations). By 7 that night the apparatus of the State had rolled over us once more and we were left with a farm which was silent apart from the odd quack. This came about because we had another "monitoring" visit from a Ministry vet (cattle left on farms are being examined by a vet at 48 hour intervals for 2 weeks). The vet today was Doris Olander, from Wisconsin. She knocked Alan into shape over the phone –I noticed he stopped making flippant remarks and started quietly saying "yes.… ………yes."
Doris thought the situation was absurd and that the cattle should go immediately as they were a "Dangerous Contact" and were not going to benefit from being left and Alan should "Get out there and make some money" (they don't care for malingerers in Wisconsin). "Do you think you can do that?" I said. Yes, she thought she could…. as she put it "I'm dogged."

They all descended on us by 4 o' clock: MAFF official, Valuer, Health and Safety Inspector, slaughterman, soldier, haulier, loader, disinfectant unit and, of course, Doris. Everyone knows their job by now and went about it efficiently. Then, at the end, Doris said "I'm going to break your husband's heart, his hams are going to have to go in the wagon, too!" During the morning visit, Alan had showed her round the butchery and explained how we cured our own hams. Doris thought, as we couldn't prove when the pigs were killed, the hams should be trashed. Ken, the slaughterman, was shocked "You can't do that !" She smiled but replied firmly, "I'm the big woman here." And, once the (rather surprised) Army had asked for and received authorization and the even more surprised haulier had asked for and received authorization, in they went.

We wonder if, when the final grim roll goes up on the internet, amongst the thousands of cattle, sheep, pigs and goats destroyed we will see "6 dry-cured hams and 2 sides of bacon."

Top of Page

Monday 14th May
It has been a funny couple of weeks. I felt it would be a relief when the four-legged animals went and only us two-legs were left. (Sorry, I forgot the dogs, but they may have their own agenda, four of them absconded and had to be rescued, at vast expense, from the Dog Pound!) In some ways it was a relief, because we knew then we wouldn't get the disease, although some parts of the farm have to be treated as "infected."

Doris (and other Ministry vets) were dubious about the poultry but "Epidemiology", when referred to, seem quite happy so I have a license to kill and sell, as it were. So we will potter on with them for a while.

On the other hand we, like others round us, seem to be going quietly mad. Alan, despite having a professional pressure washing business entirely based around cleaning agricultural premises, is unable to get a contract from the Ministry to clean sites. This is having a detrimental effect on his nerves. The Ministry has had our details from Week One so he doesn't know whether to blame God or Freemasonry, either way he's taking it personally.

I, on the other hand, should have no worries. But, in the last two weeks I have: driven away from petrol pumps without paying; left £3000 in an unlocked car overnight; stolen a head of celery from my local supermarket (I'd rather you didn't mention that last one to anyone else because I've been too embarrassed to admit to it yet). It's either early onset Alzheimer's or I'm still a bit stressed.

We are not alone, though. All around farmers are ploughing and rolling fields like mad things, planting potatoes, or anything that might grow (which isn't much, really, until Global Warming takes hold) and several have enquired about geese. As we do geese for Christmas, this is quite worrying, a county of wall to wall geese might affect the Christmas trade somewhat, but it is hard not to sympathise with farmers who just want to have something to look after. It might be hard to accept after some of the bad press, but farming as it is practised

round here, is a nurturing profession. I know your average horny-handed peasant doesn't appear to have much in common with old touchy-feely Charlie from "Casualty" but, in a livestock rearing area like this, a lot of effort goes into producing a live offspring, be it calf, pig, or lamb, with no thought to cost-effectiveness. In fact, Charlie would feel right at home in a lambing shed round here. Though he probably doesn't go down the pub with a prolapse needle stuck in his hat when his shift finishes.

This, however, does not mean that they are a unified group of people, or easy to get along with, especially under pressure. At the moment the Cumberland News is publishing a page of acknowledgements from farmers thanking friends, family, and, in many cases, MAFF officials and slaughtermen, for their support. I think in a few months we should all consider having apologies printed: "Sorry for being a bit ratty for the last few months I haven't been myself, but the police say I will get the shotgun license back any day now."

I had to go and see Head of Contracts, at the Ministry today, a man who, only last week, I wrote a nasty letter to, telling him how disgusted I was with the system. He turns out, disconcertingly, to be a very nice man who looks like the lead singer in an Eighties rock band. I tell him my problems, he tells me his. His turn out to be worse. Now there is a man who could grow to hate farmers. It seems unnecessary to identify myself as the person who wrote him an abusive letter last week. So I came home and designed a new logo for the business notepaper so he will perhaps not make the connection. Who says you can't trust farmers?

Friday 31st August
It seems a strange time to conclude a Foot and Mouth diary when no-one in this area has attempted to restock yet and with a new outbreak just announced in Northumbria. So this will have to be a "state of play" report rather than, as hoped, an epitaph.

The countryside is divided between those who have been cleared, compensated and are looking forward and those who are holed-up, half-mad and trying to operate with a Form D notice on their farms, a backlog of stock, abattoirs offering ridiculously low prices, the endless, ever-changing rules for moving livestock, vehicles, and crop,and, of course, bills the same as last year, if not higher because more animals were fed for longer this Spring.

Not surprisingly this leads to tension and ill-feeling. If you are struggling to survive and you hear there is a waiting list for new Jags in Penrith you could get to feeling a tad bitter. Still, I'm sure the resentment will wear off in a generation or two.

We are fortunate in having already diversified into contract cleaning and retailing our own meat, which luckily includes poultry, so we have had an income during this difficult time. This means I can save all my resentment for MAFF.

I was looking forward to booking my season ticket for the public enquiry that one would have assumed was inevitable after a Government Ministry had overseen a debacle on this scale. Then MAFF became DEFRA. A different name, you see, so everything will be all right now, silly! Just like when Winscale became Sellafield.

Meanwhile back in the peace and quiet of the countryside fields are filling up with what at first glance appear to be cows, but then the sunshine glints on them an you realise that they are plastic-wrapped round bales. They are like an occupying army this year because of the Grass Problem.

If you have eldery parents with a lawn you will know how they start to fret if it hasn't been mowed for a week because after two weeks it will have "got away" on them. Then imagine a farmer's feelings watching acres of burgeoning grassland with nothing to graze it. The prospect of carefully nurtured sward erupting into a tussocky wilderness can engender near panic. For a while it was the only topic of conversation : a few pleasanteries then, "What's Alan doing with his grass?" This was a tricky question, all I could say was, "He's making patterns in it." He mowed a few strips round the edges of fields, then round the odd feature, then a few up the middle, then stopped. When questioned he said it was to stop the geese getting lost, but then he started muttering about the Incas patterns being visible from Space. I'm inclined to think he is trying to make contact with his home planet.

We might be starting our clean-up next week, finally. It will be such a relief to get that finished that I find myself almost looking forward to Christmas, which is unusual when you are a turkey producer, I can assure you. It will probably be Spring before we restock with sheep, cattle and pigs. I have heard that they are going to test the sheep on the fells of the central Lake District in the Autumn. My mother says, "When they look for it they'll find it." I hope she isn't proved right but I think it is too soon to say it's over and sell the film rights.

To look on the positive side: I have been able to spend more time with the boys this summer; we have had time to think about where the business is going; writing this diary has put me back in contact with old friends in foreign parts; and we have really appreciated the expressions of concern and support we have received from so many people.
Thank you.
Marie

BBC
©MMI

BBC Radio Cumbria's web site had a comprehensive foot and mouth section. Marie Stockdale was one of four people who kept web diaries. The site increased its number of hits by 387% from February to March 2001. Another feature of the outbreak was the number of farmers who learned how to use computers!

NO ENTRY: Animal Disease Control Precautions

Caz Graham

Caz Graham was brought up on her family's farm at Cargo just north of Carlisle. She works in radio and television and produced and presented a late night foot and mouth phone-in programme for BBC Radio Cumbria during March and April.

Cargo's Magic Cows

We have magic cows on our Dad's farm at Cargo. They could be remnants from some strange mythical creatures. They're not like a small pedigree herd of phoenix; they didn't rise as great Friesian cow-gods, black and dusty and slightly surprised from any pile of ashes. They just looked into the jaws of the monstrous carnivorous fire, sniffed it with wide quivering nostrils and gave it a wide berth, tails flicking, flames reflecting back to where they came from, leaping orange in big brown eyes.

'No burning glory and resurrection for us, no compensation claims and lingering whiff of disinfectant in our fields', they murmured to each other, twice a day as they padded through the clart up the lonning and into the milking parlour. 'Not for us, those figures on the web site, the name check on Border telly. No thanks.'

Of course, they've played this game before. Back in 1967 while all their cattle neighbours turned their hooves to heaven, this lot stood firm.

So how long did they nonchalantly refuse to converse with this new updated virus?

Well, there was that brief but passionate interchange back at the start, on Black Thursday. The day no one knew where to look, who to ring, how to find out what was to be killed, what was to be saved. It felt biblical. Nick Brown seemed to be sharpening his grim scythe right outside their sheds, black cloak flapping in the wind, but then just as the sound of metal on rock faded away, he'd upped and offed like a bad lad caught filching milk from the parlour. Embarrassed guilty looks. Disclaimers. Furious farmers. Placid happy cattle, warm breath still clouding out as they poked their noses over corrugated iron shed doors in the March evening, a ground frost trying its hardest to cool us all down.

Then there was their sheer sticking power. Where did they get these skills? Day after day furnished the web site with more and more farms; Castletown, Blackford, Burgh by Sands, Beaumont, Rockcliffe, more at Burgh by Sands, more at Rockcliffe. We had our own firebreak circle – except in reverse: we were in the middle and everybody else was burning while we sat cool, as if doused in water and sand to stop the flames, a halo

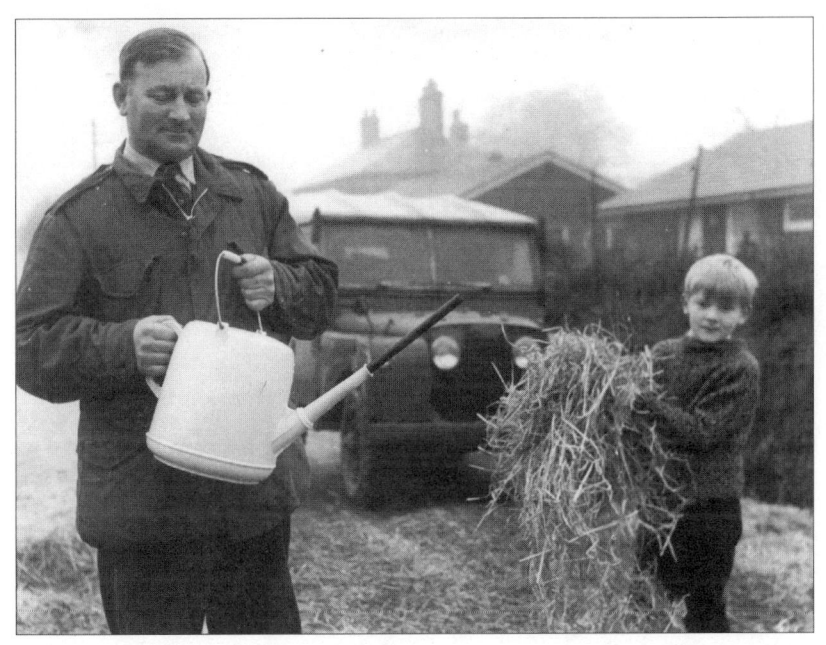

Photo: Cumberland News

William Graham with his son Robert laying straw across the road in Cargo in the 1967 outbreak.

of disinfectant shimmering around our land. Confirmed cases topped five hundred, then eight hundred, then a thousand; new lambs drowned in mud next to their mothers in fields far from their farms, the smallest death penalties signed by Restriction of Movement Orders. Stockmen spat as hefted flocks outstayed their winter resting on lowland plains, Longtown, Silloth and Wigton emptied of livestock. The sheep that had stayed on the fell farms, restless in fields they knew they should be out of, poured into wagon after wagon, and hardy shepherds wept at the waste of it all. The dismal convoys lined the roads round Great Orton, macabre cargos, half dead, half alive, all heading for the same pits.

And still Cargo's magic cows gazed innocently over their doors, impatient to be out in the fields, still breathing and crapping and being awkward buggers at milking, and doing all those other cattle things.

Week after week went by. I went on holiday, to see the sacred cows of Nepal, as well as for a spot of trekking.

'You don't know how lucky you are,' I scolded them.

'Even if you *got* foot and mouth, no one would stick a stun gun at *your* head.'

The worst they were contending with were two-inch leaches and they hardly raised an eyebrow at them either.

And when I got back home, those magic cows at Cargo were still there. I was amazed. They'd outlived nearly everything all around. They'd been within three kilometres of infected farms for more than a month and they'd breathed smoke from a pyre not half a mile away. If these beasts weren't dead yet, nothing would get them. Or so you hope for a couple of minutes while you sip your coffee before nipping out to top up the disinfectant on the straw again.

The next time they did their Houdini stuff, I'd been out interviewing at a farm on the Solway plain; a farm that looked out onto the windswept bleakness of the Solway Firth, where the air can ring with the cries of oystercatchers, the salt hangs in the air and stays on your face after, when you lick your lips, and where the spring tides creep with straying fingers of water just too close for comfort. The wind was whipping the marsh grass and gusting into the yard and all the recordings I made outside were distorted by the thick boomy disturbance of poor May weather. I'd needed a license from MAFF to go on the farm. They'd lost their pedigree Friesian dairy herd a month earlier and I was talking to them about how they were hoping to plan for the future. The future. And just when was that scheduled to start, they asked me. They hadn't even been able to start disinfecting. The administration was so stretched that even now, more than four weeks after the slaughter men had pulled off their stained white plastic overalls and walked away, three weeks after the bloated cattle had been loaded onto trucks and carted off along with their smell, still no one from MAFF had been to tell them what needed disinfecting, which buildings needed knocking down and which could stay. How can you plan for the future when you can't even get on with the present?

They'd asked how our farm was doing, how our cattle were getting along, and I was slightly embarrassed to say that we were still fine. Amazingly. It seems almost obscene when everyone else has suffered so much. But let's not knock it.

I got home, fed the interviews from my minidisc recorder into my computer, edited for half an hour and then got ready to go down to the farm to take my Mum into hospital to see her consultant. The phone rings. It's my brother-in-law.

'How soon can you get here? We've got it. We don't want to leave Mum on her own while everyone else is out with the vet.'

In the farm kitchen the vet sits at the table, white overalls, feet out of wellies in blue socks, curling under her ankles, tapping to a non-existent tune. There's hay on the carpet. She's young and Scottish and has a blond ponytail. You can imagine going to the pub with her. She's filling in forms with a blue biro that she's been chewing. The phone calls to London have already been made, the A-Notice sits burning a hole in the table. One brother sits opposite her, flattening out maps of fields, the other stands by the Aga leaning on the hot side, his face reddening. His wife sits in one comfy chair, Mum in the other, looking very grey and all of her seventy-five years. There's nothing to say, really. It's been a long time coming.

Robbie, who's two, toddles in and out of the back kitchen with his plastic cows, trailing more hay through onto the carpet. He's wearing a boiler suit like his Dad's. He puts some of his cattle in Mum's tumble-dryer. This is his favourite game.

'Cows in for milking now', he beams at us all. He pulls the sliding door shut, with great effort, leaving himself alone to concentrate on working his plastic dairy herd.

A different vet who'd been called for a second opinion comes in the back door.

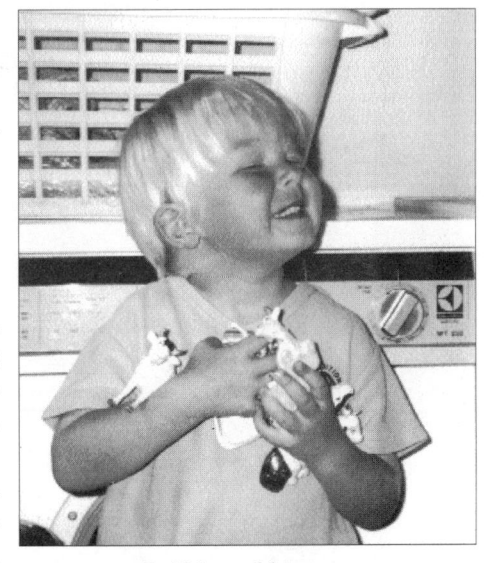

Robbie and his cows

He's Scottish too, older, wiry, and not at all happy. He brushes off offers of coffee, shaking his head.

'I don't understand why these cattle are still alive.'

Nor do we really, we thought they'd have gone weeks ago.

The back kitchen door makes strange noises then slides open. Robbie peers through.

'Tanker's late today' he says.

'Is it Robbie? Well you'll just have to wait for it then. Have you got all them cattle milked yet?' his Dad asks.

The vet continues.

'The whole herd should have gone down with it by now if these lacerations we're looking at have been caused by foot and mouth. They're ten days old and they've all but healed.'

He wants to inspect the rest of the stock. Everything on the farm.

But whatever happens we're certain that this is the end. We've got the A-Notice and London have us clocked. Even if it all turns out to be a ghastly mistake there's no way these faceless voices down south will reprieve us.

The pile of coffee cups by the sink grows and I take Mum to hospital.

Ministry of Agriculture, Fisheries and Food
National Assembly for Wales Agriculture Department

Animal Health Act 1981
Foot-and-Mouth Disease Order 1983 (Articles 5 and 9)

FORM A - Notice declaring infected place

To: MESSERS W. H. GRAHAM
of: CARGO FARM, CARGO, CARLISLE, CA6 4EW.

I, the undersigned, being (*Delete as appropriate)

- *a police constable
- *an inspector of the Ministry of Agriculture, Fisheries and Food
- *an inspector of the local authority for the _____ of _____

hereby give you notice as the occupier of the undermentioned premises that in accordance with the provisions of the above order the **undermentioned premises** are hereby declared to be an **infected place** for the purposes of the said order and that the premises accordingly become subject to the Rules specified in this notice which are printed on the back hereof. Any infringement of these rules may constitute an offence against the Animal Health Act 1981 and render a person liable to heavy penalties on conviction.

This notice remains in force until it is withdrawn by a subsequent notice (Form B) served on you by a Veterinary Inspector.

Description of infected place, stating parish where applicable, district/borough and county+

Premises: CARGO FARM.
Parish: ROSE KINGMOOR.
District/borough+: CARLISLE
County: CUMBRIA

+ in Scotland insert name of regional or islands council

Signed: Helen F Buchanan   Date: 18/5/01
Name in BLOCK LETTERS: HELEN F. BUCHANAN.
Official address: MAFF CARLISLE, HADRIAN HOUSE, CARLISLE

NOTE: The police constable or inspector is with all practicable speed to send copies of this notice to the Divisional Veterinary Manager, to the local authority, to the police officer in charge of the nearest operational police station of the police force for the area, and to the Veterinary Exotic Diseases Team, Head Office, Ministry of Agriculture, Fisheries and Food, 1A Page Street, London SW1P 4PQ.

FM 30 (3/01)

We watch the other patients and read about stricken farmers in the Cumberland News while we're waiting to see the hip man, and I try to talk about anything except bad hips and foot and mouth. I don't succeed for very long. The consultant, however, is at least a diversion and he has inconclusive news rather than bad so that feels like a positive result. But it is, of course, only killing time before we go home for the killing. We head back through the Friday evening rush hour traffic. As we pull closer to the village, along the new road, we're passed by an army Land Rover coming in the opposite direction. Must be ours. Must have forgotten something.

My mobile rings. Lisa, my sister-in-law. Excited. More than excited.

'They've gone! They say we haven't got it and they're not going to kill anything, anything at all! They've scrapped the A-Notice. They've given us a B-Notice, whatever that is.'

Ministry of Agriculture, Fisheries and Food
National Assembly for Wales Agriculture Department
Animal Health Act 1981
Foot-and-Mouth Disease Order 1983 (Articles 5 and 6)

FORM B - Withdrawal of notice declaring infected place (Form A)

To: MESSERS GRAHAM

of: CARGO FARM
CARGO
CARLISLE.

I, the undersigned, being a veterinary inspector of the Ministry of Agriculture, Fisheries and Food hereby withdraw, as from

this 18TH day of MAY 2001.

The infected Place Notice (Form A) signed by HELEN BUCHANAN and served on you on the 18TH day of MAY 2001

and any other Notice which may have been served on you by a veterinary inspector altering the limits of the infected place.

Signed: Helen F Buchanan   Date: 18/5/01

Name in BLOCK LETTERS: HELEN F. BUCHANAN.

Official address: MAFF CARLISLE,
HADRIAN HOUSE
CARLISLE.

NOTE: The veterinary inspector is with all practicable speed to send copies of this notice to the Divisional Veterinary Manager, to the local authority, to the police officer in charge of the nearest operational police station of the police force for the area, and to the Veterinary Exotic Diseases Team, Head Office, Ministry of Agriculture, Fisheries and Food, 1A Page Street, London SW1P 4PQ.

We can't believe it. We can't stop grinning. Huge manic grins. Still driving, I ring my brother-in-law.

'Have you heard? We haven't got it now! It was a mistake and they're not going to shoot anything! I know. It's crazy.'

None of us believe it.

As we pull into the drive the vets are outside in the yard washing down their boiler suits and wellies. There are four new people who've arrived since we left for the hospital. Two epidemiologists and two valuers.

Lisa explains that the second vet is convinced that the lacerations they'd discovered in the mouths of four cattle couldn't have been caused by foot and mouth; they were already healing and too old, the rest of the cattle should be severely ill. The cuts must have come from something else; perhaps they'd been chewing a door with a sharp edge, perhaps there'd been some wire in the straw they'd been feeding on. But whatever, they shouldn't have to die. These cattle had set up a sophisticated hoax, obviously for a kind of bovine laugh, and had only just been found out. Bacon saved, as it were, to mix our farmyard metaphors. Ten minutes later eight slaughter men arrive. And then leave again.

Now it's June. The sun is blasting down with uncharacteristic enthusiasm. The heat makes itself comfortable and decides to set up home in the bottom fields down by the river and the grass is as high as a small calf's eye. They wallow in buttercups, and every type of meadow grass you can imagine, nostrils just sticking out over the top of this green and yellow and purple blanket, luxuriating in their bed-cum-restaurant of sorrel and clover. No other cattle for miles. Magic cows. No other explanation.

NO ENTRY: Animal Disease Control Precautions

John Darwell

John Darwell is an independent photographer specialising in global, industrial and environmental issues. His work has been exhibited and published widely both nationally and internationally and is included in a number of major collections including the Victoria and Albert Museum, London and the Metropolitan Museum of Art, New York. His latest book 'Legacy' is a view inside the 30 km exclusion zone that surrounds the power plant at Chernobyl. He is aiming to publish a book of photographs recording the foot and mouth crisis in Cumbria, provisionally entitled 'Dark Days' within the next year.

When I was asked to write a piece for this book the thing that came to mind was a series of events and moments that I experienced whilst documenting what was taking place in Cumbria during the first seven months of 2001. The actual sequence of events has blurred in terms of sequence but I have tried here to put across something of the atmosphere of the time.

February

My first experience of foot and mouth. Contacted by a friend living in the Eden Valley who declared 'John, we really should be doing something about this. There are farmers going down all around me here. Someone should be recording what's happening!'

For a long time I agonised over whether or not I should get involved. I felt like an ambulance-chaser going out to photograph people's misery and anguish. Articles on the TV and radio talked of farmers crying by the roadside as their flocks and herds were culled. This was too close for me. I have photographed environmental disasters all around the world, but this was on my doorstep, places I drove past on a regular basis, relatives succumbing to the disease. How could I possibly photograph this?

I decided if I was to photograph what was happening the work would have to be non-intrusive. I didn't want pictures of crying farmers or bolt guns in action, but rather I would photograph what I saw whilst driving around the lanes of Cumbria, the sights everyone could see.

My friend phoned me back a week later, 'John, there's nothing left around here. It's too depressing. I don't want to get involved.' I started to venture out to see what was taking place; men in white suits everywhere, a tangible sense of paranoia everywhere I went. It was very hard to get out of the car to take photographs, people's reactions were unpredictable and emotions were understandably running high.

March

Driving through Eden Valley, 'Closed' and 'Keep Out' signs everywhere. Drove past a field piled high with dead sheep. Approached two men working in the field and asked if I could take some shots from the road. After a while they invited me into the field. 'Do you know there are over a thousand sheep there. They belong to my brother-in-law. He won't come out of the farmhouse 'til it's all over. All my stock went last week. Do you know, if you look across the valley there's not one sheep left on any farm'. I spoke to the ministry vet on site about what I was doing and he said he'd speak to MAFF on my behalf. That night he phoned to say that 'under no circumstances were MAFF prepared to let me photograph what they were doing'.

I spoke to the County Council regarding a letter of support which would've helped in terms of people understanding that I wasn't a press photographer just out for a good photo, but rather someone who was trying to show what was happening because it was important from a historical point of view. Call came back to say the County wouldn't help me because 'they don't want Cumbria associated with foot and mouth!' which was fairly ironic seeing that every time you turned on the TV news or looked at a paper there we were in all our gory glory. Phrases like 'head in sand' sprang to mind!

Went up Hartside. From the top looking towards Penrith you could see nine fires burning. Driving back down the hill, passed farmyard full of dead pigs. The guys standing around didn't look like they'd take kindly to me stopping. Stopped in Langwathby to photograph 'Voluntary Road Closure' sign in village. Farmer ran across road to ask what I was doing, when I explained he replied: 'Thank goodness someone is showing what's happening', a phrase I was about to hear over and over again.

Followed two wagons full of live sheep on their way to Great Orton. Driving around back roads near Ivegill, no one about, passing piles of dead sheep, 'Keep Out' everywhere, Tony Blair on radio insisting 'the countryside is open for business', me thinking 'not round here it ain't mate!'

April

Things continuing pretty much the same, fires everywhere, closing bedroom windows at night to keep smell of pyres out. Army everywhere, feels like state of siege. Can't move in Tesco's cafe for camouflage uniforms. Watch removal of cow carcasses from farm opposite my friend's window.

Driving along A6 can see huge fire in distance. Follow it to Welton. Smoke obliterating Caldbeck. Pyre right beside road, smoke turning day into night. Talk to farmer who declares: 'I'm glad you're photographing this as no one would believe it otherwise!'

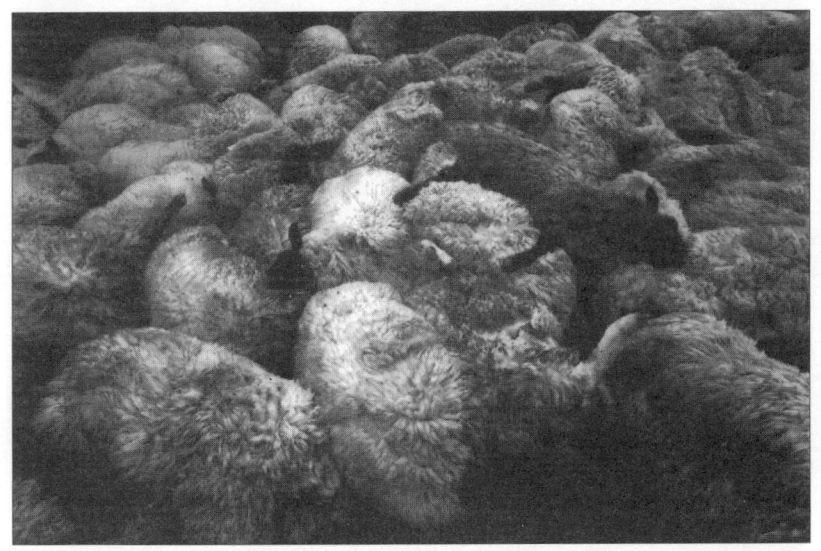

Thousand dead sheep, Eden

Photo: John Darwell

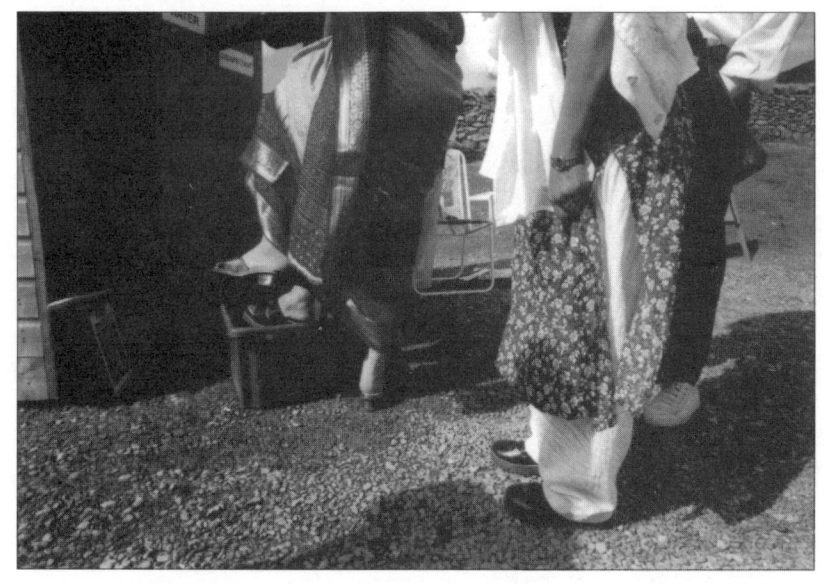

Photo: John Darwell

Bangladeshi teacher trainers on a first visit to Cumbria going through the disinfecting process before walking on the fells

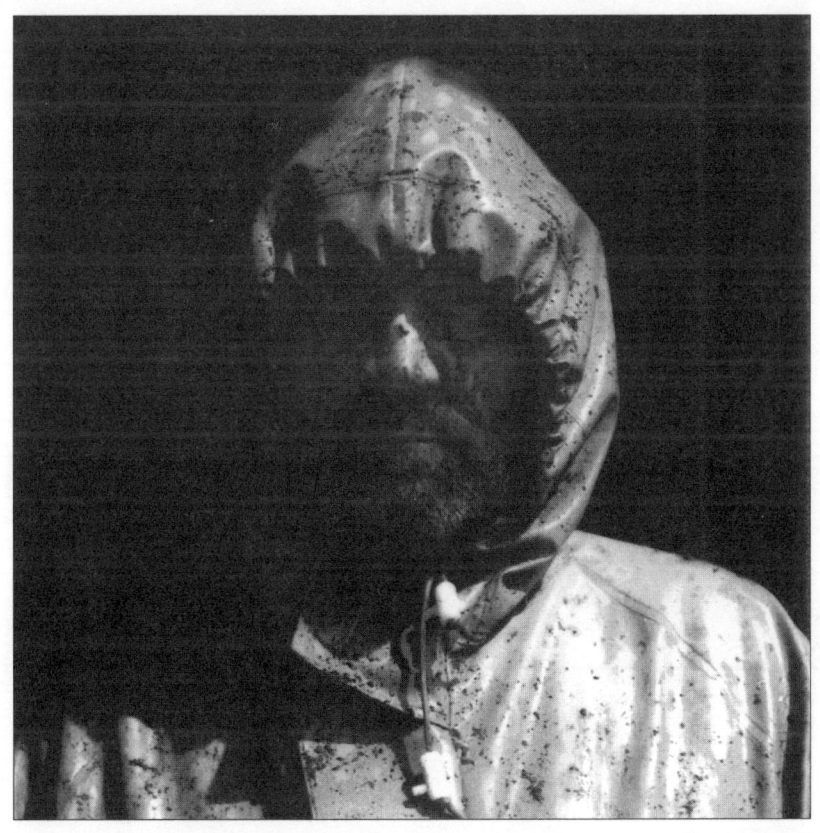

Photo: John Darwell

Robert after pressure washing cattle shed roof

Get permission to photograph the clean-up on three farms. Teams of men in cherry pickers up in the roofs of cattle sheds de-greasing, guys in full respirator gear ripping asbestos roofing out of milking parlours, everywhere frenetic activity. Many of the men are farmers; shepherds and cowmen who had lost stock now working for MAFF. I photograph the clean-up over the next few weeks; de-grease, pull down, disinfect. MAFF inspector returns and fails the work. Now all concrete barriers in cattle sheds need removing and plaster from walls, then repeat of disinfecting process.

Continue photographing on farms and around county, the radio declares that due to health concerns burning will now stop. Over next few days I count eleven new fires.

May/June

On 'my farms' work continues, ripping out and burning all wooden feed troughs, cutting out wooden barn doors, removing hardcore from farmyard. Job seems endless. MAFF changes the rules, not for first time! This leaves farmers confused and angry. MAFF will no longer pay for 'betterment' on farms, which is odd as it's MAFF inspectors who are insisting on the work being done.

MAFF becomes DEFRA – bit like Windscale becoming Sellafield: different name same old story! Rules changed again, now no cleaning needs to be done above ten feet. Is this down to scientific advice or economics? I have my view!

Fells reopen for limited access. I photograph walkers queuing up to stand in disinfectant buckets. Farmers not happy at this development fearing spread of disease to previously untouched areas.

July

Still driving around, still 'closed' signs everywhere and more new cases in the paper every week. Listening to national news you'd think it was all over. We've become the forgotten county! Five cases in Thirsk make news headlines, thirteen new cases in Cumbria – nothing. Work on farms continues apace but can sense everyone's getting really fed up and disillusioned.

August

Tony Blair calls halt to clean up due to expense and I'm still taking pictures.

I would like to thank Ian and Celia at Littoral without whose enthusiastic support none of the aforementioned photographic work would have been possible.

Colin Shelbourn

Colin Shelbourn is a writer and cartoonist. He lives near Kendal. As well as producing books, educational material and cards, he has a regular slot in the Westmorland Gazette. Throughout the foot and mouth crisis he supplied some much needed light relief. You can see several of his cartoons throughout the book as well as the two below.

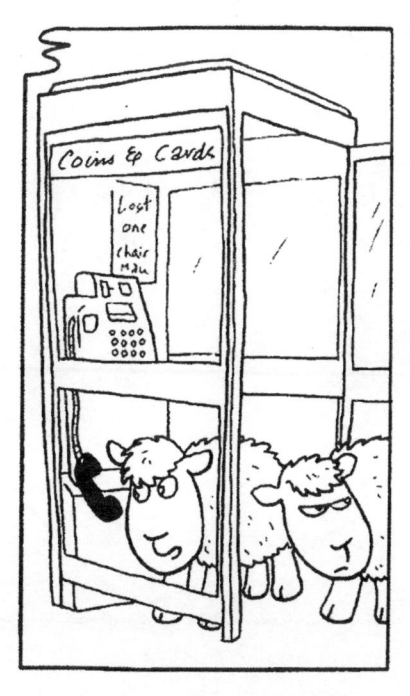

"Brewery Theatre? Do you have any pantomime calf costumes for hire?"

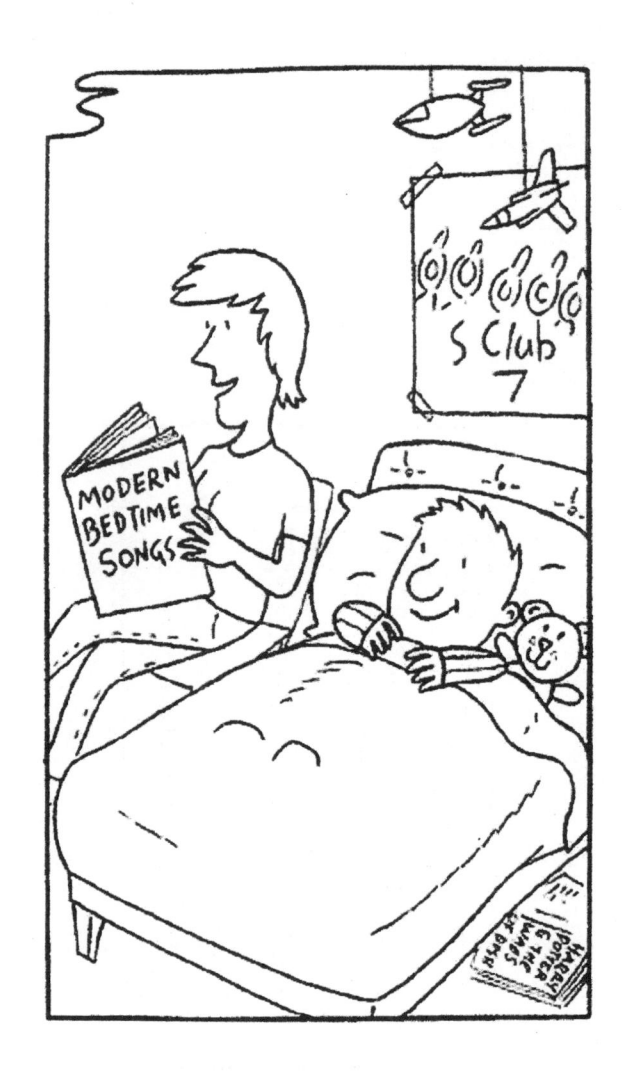

"Old MacDonald had a
bio-security intensification
zone, ei ei oh"

Hunter Davies

Hunter Davies was brought up in Carlisle. He is a writer and broadcaster and has written many books about his native Cumbria. He now lives near Loweswater with his wife, the writer Margaret Forster.

One of the ways I'll remember 2001 will be foot and mouth. One of the ways I'll remember 2001's foot and mouth will be my 2001 foot and mouth memorabilia.

I started collecting the notices around May, just for my own amusement, as I wandered on the local roads from our house at Loweswater.

I realised there were so many of them, put up by different bodies, such as the National Park, Cumbria County Council, the National Trust. Some were home made, written by farmers themselves. Some were printed by farm magazines, such as 'Farmers Guardian', given out to readers. Some were pretty, with little vignettes and drawings.

I also noticed a chronological sequence to them, as the disease got more serious. In the early weeks, the notices were polite, announcing a voluntary ban. As it went on, the notices became heavier with convoluted legalese.

I didn't actually steal the notices. Just took photographs of them. But as the weeks went on, I asked local farmers to give me any copies they might be about to chuck out. One day I met a volunteer who was going around putting up new ones and she kindly gave

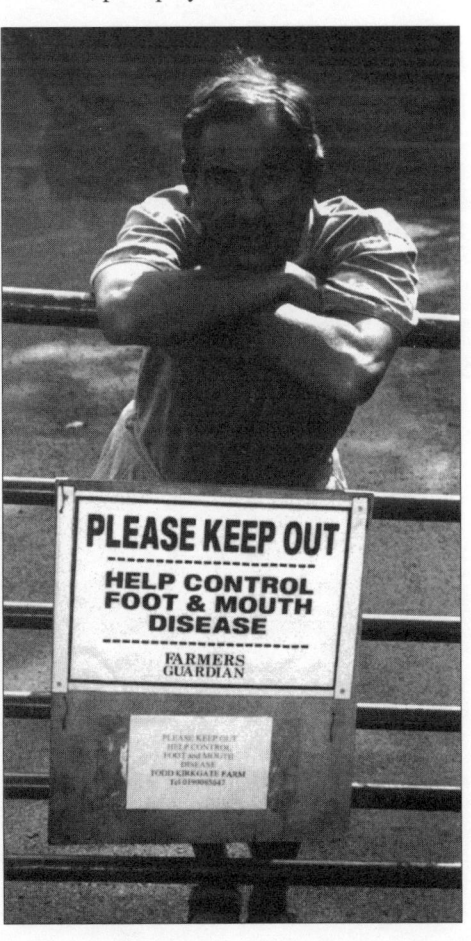

> **Cumbria**
> COUNTY COUNCIL
>
> **Due to Foot and Mouth restrictions please use the temporary diversion and follow the waymarks.**
>
> Thank you
> Cumbria County Council

me a spare one.

I made regular visits to our local tourist office in Cockermouth, and those in Keswick, Whitehaven and Maryport, picking up any leaflets or notices to do with foot and mouth. I also cut out articles from the Cumberland News. Their foot and mouth coverage has been excellent. It's all a bit daft really. As if I hadn't got enough rubbish, I mean treasures.

At any one moment, I have about twenty collections on the go, which include Beatles memorabilia, football books and programmes, Prime Ministers's autographs, suffragette post cards, first editions of newspapers and magazines.

A lot of my collections are to do with Cumbria, such as Beatrix Potter books, Lake District post cards, Lake District guide books, cheques from dead Cumbrian banks, letter heads from old Cumbrian shops and businesses. So local foot and mouth stuff fitted in with my Cumbrian collections generally.

It's a disease, collecting, and usually it begins with an inability to throw anything out. You start as an accumulator, then realise you have acquired and kept or not thrown out certain related items, so you decide to go on and add to them.

I kept for example some of Carlisle United's home programmes for the 1974-75 season, that wondrous season when they were in the First Division, blink and you missed it. I've only now just finished collecting every one, buying them from dealers or stalls or garage sales.

Some of my collections are done because I

> **Lake District**
> National Park Authority
>
> 立入厳禁
> 口蹄疫
>
> 現在、この道の通行は法律で禁止されています。
> ※ 最高罰金額5千ポンド
>
> 口蹄疫は、田園地帯の住民の生活を脅かす家畜伝染病であるため、丘陵、農地、森林地を通る歩行者道、乗馬道は、全て、一般の使用を許可されていません。
>
> より詳しい情報をお求めの方は
> 0845-6014-068まで

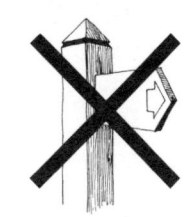

This japanese notice became a collector's item!

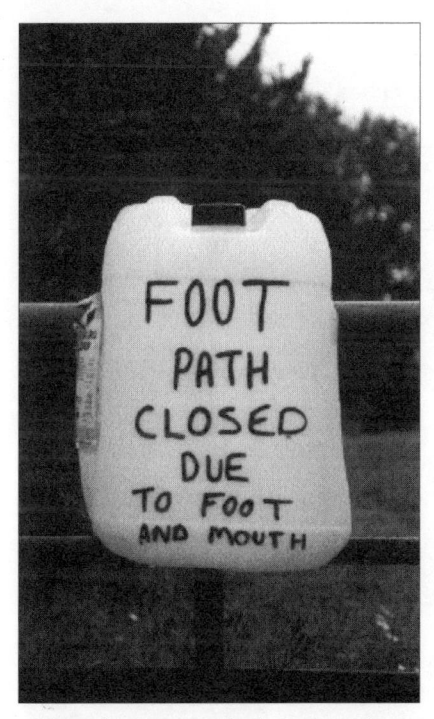

Many farmers made their own signs like this one near Red Dial, Wigton.

think they are part of our social history, such as the National Lottery. I bought a ticket on day one, Saturday November the 19th, 1994, because I wanted to have a ticket which said 'First Day Issue'. I then picked up the various leaflets during the rest of that first year. I'm not sure where they are now, but I like to think it's all historic stuff.

Collecting foot and mouth memorabilia has been social history, with political and economic overtones. Oh yes. While collecting this year's outpourings, I've been looking around for any foot and mouth memorabilia from 1967. Someone must have kept the bits and pieces. But I've never seen any. I would like to be able to compare what happened in 1967, what the notices said in our local area, compared with 2001.

When I started collecting the 2001 notices, I thought I was on my own, that I was the first person to have thought of this mad idea. Then in the Cockermouth tourist office, a girl behind the counter, who was a student on vacation, said that at her university, Nottingham, they were working on a project in the Media Studies department to compare and contrast the different notices from 1967 and 2001. I was quite pleased by that. I realised I was not alone.

But as with all collections, I had in the end to draw a line, to define what it was I thought I was doing. One of my local farming friends asked me if I'd like his copy of a ten minute government video he'd just been sent, telling him how to disinfect his farm. He said he should have had it three months ago, now it was too late, so he was going chuck it out, unless I wanted it.

No thanks, I said. I'm only collecting foot and mouth paper memorabilia. I don't do foot and mouth video. That way true madness lies...

John Malone

John (Jock) Malone from Ambleside manned one of the 34 designated fell access points which were set up by Cumbria County Council to maintain biosecurity on the high fells. The access points were in operation from the 9th of June to the 31st of July and hundreds of thousands of walkers passed through them in an effort to try to reduce the risk of spreading the disease.

Last day at Pelter Bridge – 31st July 2001
'Do I have to do both feet?'
'Only if you plan on using both feet Sir.'
This last day at the Pelter Bridge fell access point near Rydal is much the same as any other but with an added element of irony. Here we are asking people to disinfect their feet today because of the small chance that they may carry the foot and mouth virus on their boots, but tomorrow it will be safe.

Absurd as it is, most people have been extremely accommodating and do their bit, dipping their feet without complaint. The procedure, for those readers not fortunate enough to have experienced it, is to remove all mud and dust in the first tub of water and detergent, rinse off in the tub of water and then disinfect in the tub of 500:1 citric acid.

The questions are more or less the same every day:
'Why do we have to do this on the way off the fell as well as on the way on?'
'Because we don't know if those sheep have the virus and we don't want anyone taking anything nasty home.'
'Why can't we take our dogs?'
'Because we can't disinfect their feet in the citric acid and because they may scare the sheep off their normal patch. We want to keep animal to animal contact to a minimum.'
'What's the point of all this? I've just walked

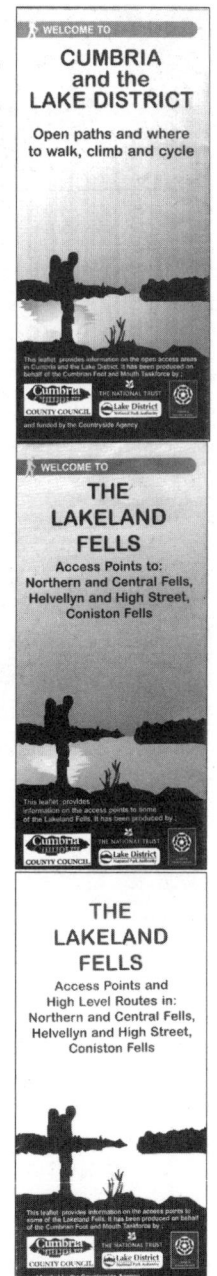

through a field of cows and there's not a disinfection tub in sight.'

'Hmmm. No system is perfect. We do what we can.'

The system was indeed imperfect. There were a great many weak points in the perimeter where people could sneak on to the fells with their dogs, and they did. Herdwick sheep are hardy creatures and apparently it's hard to tell when they have the virus. In the case of the cows, however, they would show unmistakable signs of infection so if they haven't got it then the sheep haven't.....or so we hope.

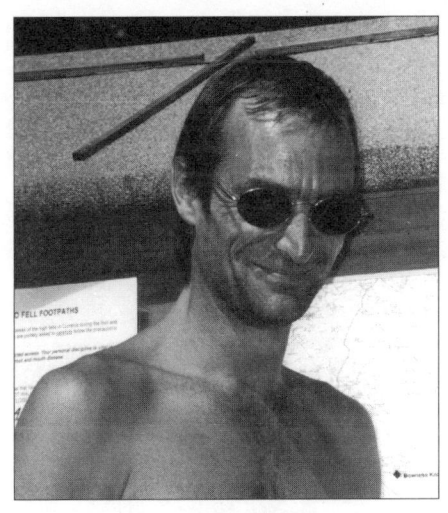

John outside his hut

Trying to explain to people why they had to go through all this fuss just for a walk was difficult at first but as the days progressed it became easier,

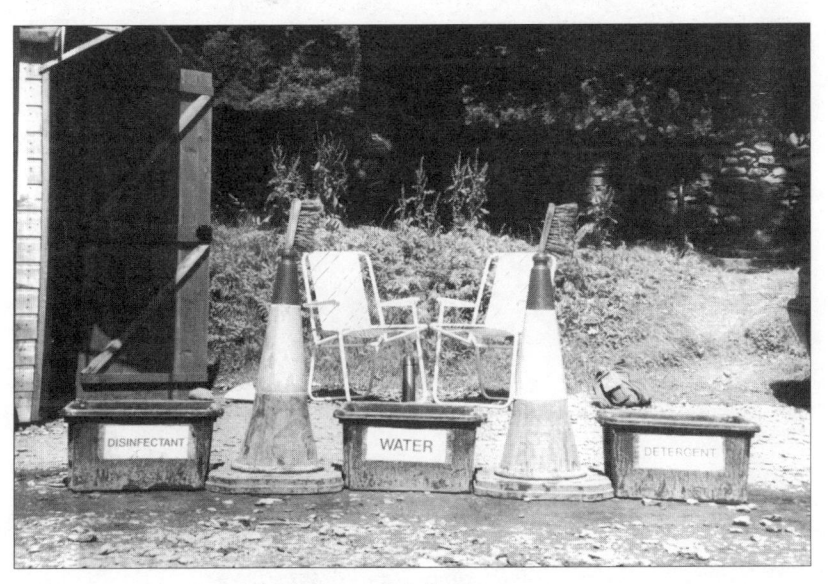

The 3-stage disinfection process

and myself and my colleagues developed a set of stock answers. After all, the questions were more or less the same every day. Towards the last day we actually started believing our own spin.

'Are you getting paid to get that suntan?'

'I work in the rain as well Ma'am.'

Ten hours a day to watch the weather taught me a little bit about mountain meteorology. Under certain conditions the mountains can make their own clouds. As the air comes off the mountain and down the leeward side it expands and its pressure drops. This can just tip the balance and cause clouds to dissolve. On one day a northerly wind off High Pike, Fairfield displayed just this behavior and a permanent hole of blue sky was above the Rydal Valley all day, yet with clouds on all horizons. Just the type of thing one notices when stuck in an open air, country car park ten hours a day.

'Is this the way to Whinlatter Pass?'

'Wrong car park, sorry Sir.'

We were more than just disinfection supervisors, we were also country guides. Many folks expressed their gratitude for our advice on directions.

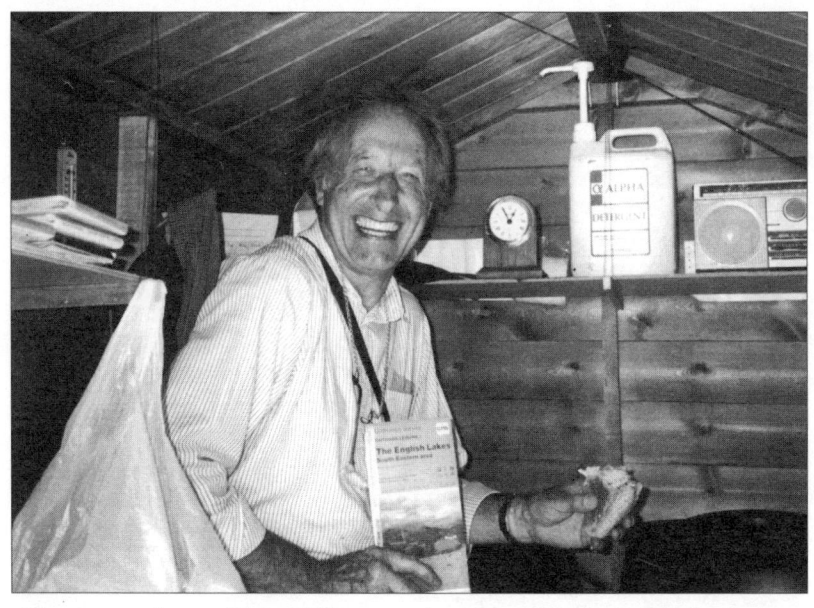

Home sweet home. Richard Kevan in the access point hut at Pelter Bridge where he built shelves and fitted a carpet.
One access point hut even got its own postal address!

Luckily most people at the access points had a good knowledge of the area. This helped quite a few walkers, guiding them to scenic routes that they may never have found otherwise.

It may have also saved the lives of a middle-aged couple who asked me how to go round the Fairfield Horseshoe. No water, no food, no proper clothing and no sense. The day was fine but in two hours it was due to change with clouds coming below the one thousand foot mark. My response to their question – 'Don't even think about it mate.'

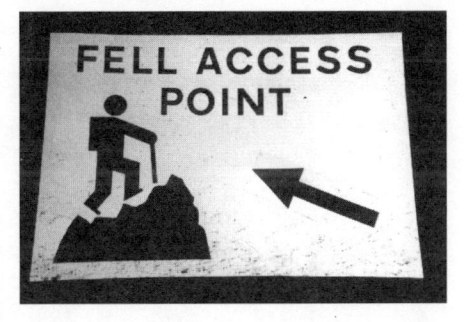

'Do you think it's a good idea to open the fells up tomorrow?'

'I don't know Sir. I just hope it's not a mistake. I don't want to see a pyre in this valley.'

Right now we're not sure about the sheep. Could they have it? Have they had it and recovered? Will they get it? We'll just have to wait and see when they finally test them. We may also find out whether or not our efforts were worthwhile. If walkers and dogs can transmit the virus then maybe we caught the one that would have otherwise got away. If they can't, then the whole thing was a waste of time and money; a point often brought up by the more cynical of our clients.

'Who pays for all this?'

'You do.' or 'We're employed by an agency on behalf of the County Council.' as appropriate.

The Council sent a water wagon every day to top us up with water and citric acid. A small part of what became a routine. Tom from Systems Recruitment, the employment agency, was the only unpredictable thing about it, his visits being at random to make sure that all the stations were properly run. The people were more sheep-like: virtually none from eight until ten, then cars arriving in unmanageable droves from ten until four, on the dot, every day, and then a near empty car park at six. The rhythm of modern life. I hope people really did use those tubs of disinfectant that we left out overnight.

At least at the end of the day, this last day at Pelter Bridge, we have some sense of having done our bit. During our stay in the car park the car crime went down to zero during working hours. Now that's a result.

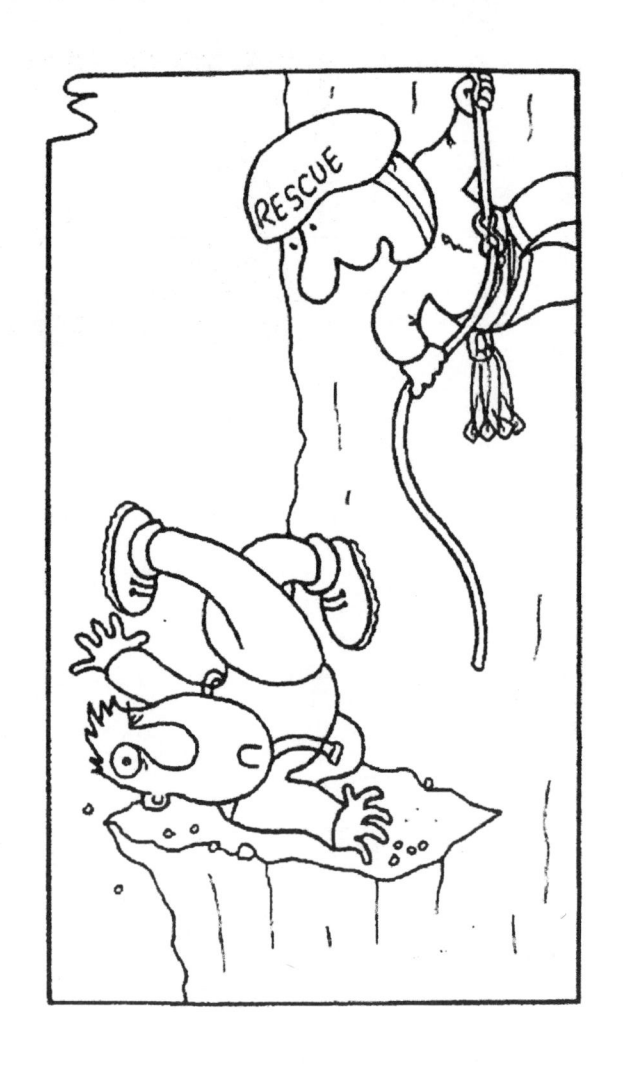

"You're lucky - this is an approved falling off point."

Deborah Cowin

Deborah Cowin owns The Necessary Angel Gallery in Keswick and designs and makes jewellery. She is a founder member and spokesperson for Cumbria Crisis Alliance, a self-help group for business people who have been badly affected by the foot and mouth outbreak.

March 21st 2001

Cumbria Crisis Alliance is only 7 days old and here we are, about to do our first rally: the Job Centre Queue. I'm 42 years old and I've never been on a demonstration before, never mind coming up with the idea and organising it! What if nobody comes? It's sleeting and cold. Andrew Bomford is here from 'PM' on Radio 4 – not having a telly, I set great store by the radio, so he's more than welcome. The final run-through for the committee goes well. Everyone has a job to do, queue organising, banners, media contacts, police liaison, coffee and tea supplies for all the journalists we hope will arrive as well as the 'Queuers'.

Half an hour before the demo kicks-off and Pack Horse Court is heaving with journalists. BBC radio and TV, ITN, ITV, Sky News, CNN,

The CNN reporter

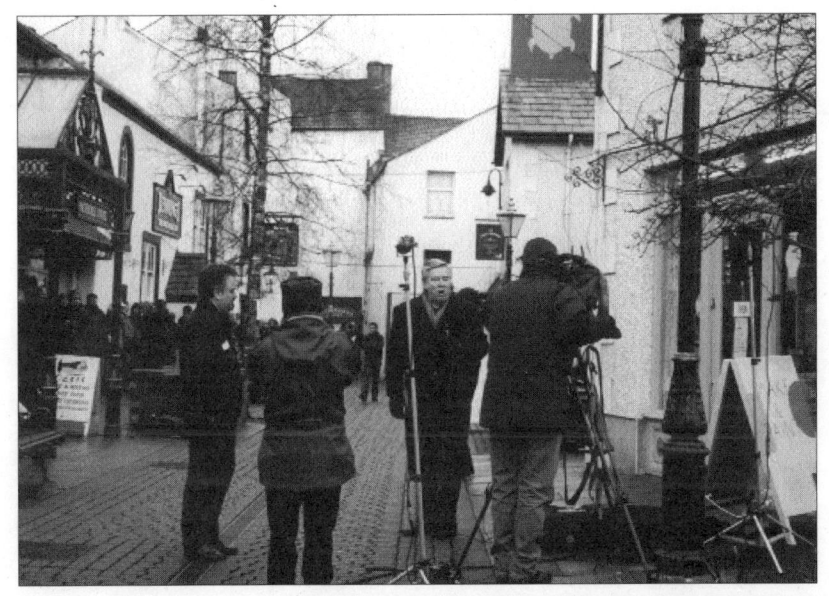

Photo: Keith James, Keswick Reminder

all the national papers (even 'The Sun', though it's too cold for topless babes today!) and international media everywhere. What if there are more journalists than us? Deep breaths, calm thoughts.

They're here! More and more people are joining the queue! I can't believe it! They're huddling under umbrellas, wrapped up in fleeces, drinking coffee, anything to stay warm. The journalists descend like hungry wolves, devouring the anger and frustration of desperate people who just don't know what the future holds for them. Various estimates of the length of the queue are given out as gospel by the anchormen looking earnestly into their cameras to tell the world of our plight. Journos rove up and down the queue, jotting people's misery down in spidery shorthand. Nobody likes the guy from the 'Daily Mail', wanting to put words into peoples' mouths. 'Can I quote you as saying.........?'

Disaster strikes CNN. Their $45,000 state-of-the-art Japanese TV camera blows over – but never mind, in true American fashion, they just get another one out of their van! The show must go on!

Someone points out Kevin Bouquet (BBC Radio 4 'PM' programme turned TV news) and I have to go and shake his hand and tell him what a big fan I am – on the RADIO! He actually looks a little bashful. Andrew

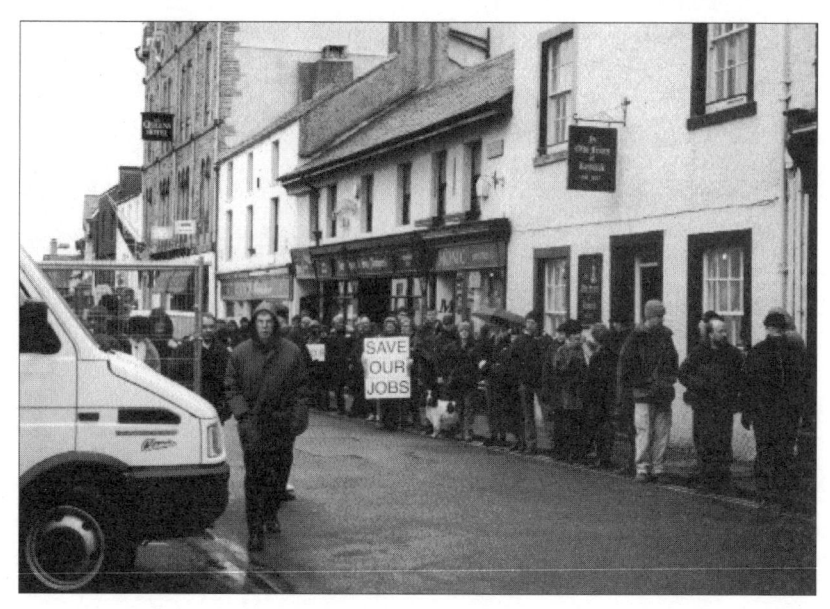

Photo: Keith James, Keswick Reminder

The queue snakes through Keswick

Bomford is still with us capturing candid comments from everybody in a very quiet way. He has to dash off soon to get the story squirted down the line for 'The World at One'.

The photographers have taken all the pictures they need so all our valiant 'Queuers' are congregating in Pack Horse Court for the group shots. John Walker jumps up onto the raised flower beds and gives everyone a big heartfelt thank you for turning out to 'queue for your jobs'. The journalists swarm into the gallery to drink hot coffee. I try and drum up some local business. Shirley from Sky News wants a new fleece so I point her in the direction of Needle Sports. Let's hope some good comes of this.

Andrew stays with us for the rest of the day and we listen to 'PM' in the gallery. When we get home friends ring us from Washington DC, San Diego, Hawaii, Tokyo all saying the same thing: 'We saw you on the telly!'

June 7th 2001

Here we are at 10 Downing Street on Election Day, me, John Walker, Terry Franks and Simon McCrum, the Alliance lawyer. We've had our meeting, we've been in the Cabinet Room, we've had a bit of a tour and while they go to the gents I'm waiting in the entrance hall. It's full of antique furniture, gorgeous flower arrangements, beautiful paintings on the wall, the smell of polished wood and there's Leo's buggy under the hall table. A door bursts open and the three of them come clattering through. Simon McCrum is in seventh heaven – 'I've pissed in the same urinal as Winston Churchill!' Sigh!

July 26th 2001

Joy Harrison from the Swan and I arrive at Rheged to do some TV interviews while we all wait for Tony Blair to arrive. I've tried to give Joy the benefit of my experience of journalists during the last 4 months but she's still feeling nervous. I smile and say hello to the TV technicians who I've come to recognise. I usher Joy off to mingle with the 'paper people'. I do my piece with Shirley from Sky News and we have a chat about how much she enjoyed her holiday with her daughter at the Leathes Head Hotel in Borrowdale. (At least we drummed up some business for someone.) I talk to CFM and 'The Independent'. I think journalism must be 99% hanging around waiting for things to happen then 1% of absolute frenzy! I'd rather be in the gallery any day. Suddenly there's a disturbance in the main journo pack. I hear someone shout 'There she is!' and there's a lot of pointing in the general direction of ....me!

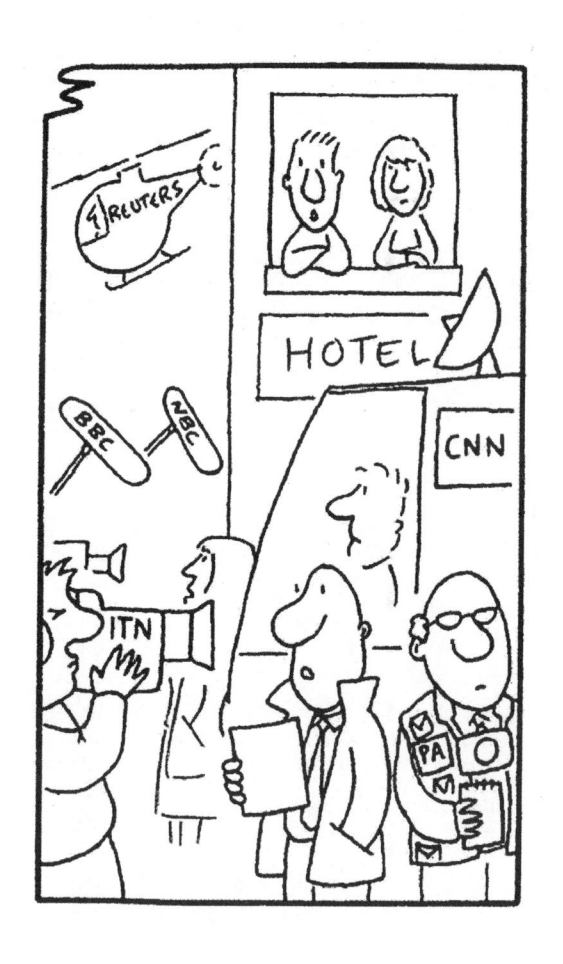

"On the other hand, visitor figures are up ....."

Martin Rushton

Martin Rushton and his wife Josie run the Bridge House Hotel in Grasmere.

April 2nd is a day that sticks in the mind. It was Monday morning and we walked through the front door of the hotel to find that there had been three cancellations. Guests had been cancelling left right & centre, ever since FMD struck in February, and yet March trade had held up remarkably well, because of our 'regulars'. But these three cancellations were different - they were large group bookings (£25K's worth) - all in May. In one morning we had seen virtually the whole of May's bookings wiped out!

Later the same week our Marketing Advisor came to tell us officially how the hotel was performing. In April we would normally expect to generate 25 to 30 bookings a week. Eric told us that we were doing just that, but this time it was minus 25 to 30!

Also that week, road signs began to appear telling people to keep away from minor roads. Joel Rasbash (our brother-in-law) had designed fifteen tarmac walks in the Lake District and we had been persuading our guests not to cancel by telling them they could walk the hills on tarmac. One of our marketing leaflets features the words 'Walk upon England's Mountains Green' taken from Blake's 'Jerusalem'. Needless to say, when FMD struck, we crossed out the 'Mountains Green' and wrote in 'Tarmac Black'. Now, it seemed, even tarmac was off-limits! We wrote to Cumbria County Council, along with one or two others, and the signs were removed. But not before many visitors had been turned away.

Day by day our hotel was haemorrhaging business at such a rate that we

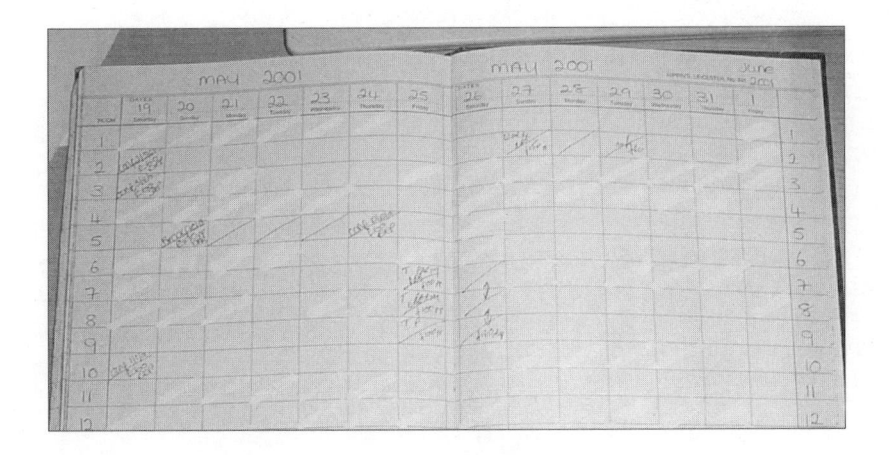

Bridge House Chronicle
Special Edition
THE LATEST NEWS FROM GRASMERE'S PREMIER HOTEL

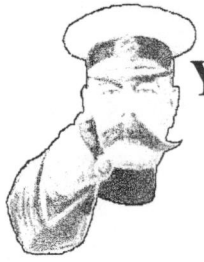

YOUR COUNTRYSIDE NEEDS YOU !

Dear Friends,
The Foot & Mouth Disease has hit the British Countryside very hard. It is harming all of the businesses & livelihoods in our area too.

However, we are circulating this, the first serious edition of the Chronicle, just to tell you why you should still come to Grasmere this Spring.

There are still lots of things to do in the Lakes, and we have listed a variety of choices overleaf. Also, we have assembled fifteen walks on quiet tarmac which still allow you to be arrested by the breathtaking scenery (as opposed to by the Local Constabulary).

So, to take advantage of our 3 night breaks this May, telephone 015394 35425 - we'd really love to see you.

Best Wishes,

From Everyone at the Bridge House Hotel in Grasmere.

Bridge House Hotel Church Bridge Grasmere Cumbria LA22 9SN
Tel 015394 35425
www.bridgehousegrasmere.co.uk

were afraid to answer the telephone. Jayne, Claire and our other staff looked at me & my wife Josie every day. They looked at us without saying a word but their eyes were constantly asking the questions, 'Is my job safe?' 'Am I going to have to find somewhere else to live?' The hotel reservations diary began to weigh a ton from all the Tippex we had used in wiping out people's bookings. I wish we'd bought shares in that company before FMD struck (and in MAFF disinfectant too!).

We set about saving the business and decided to target May with a rescue operation. Our database of 'repeat & recommend' customers is one of our key assets and we carry out mass mailings twice a year to keep guests informed & up to date about the hotel. We have about 8000 names & addresses to call on, so we sent out the 'Your Countryside Needs You' leaflets featuring discounted three night breaks. We promoted our tarmac walks and hoped that people would be persuaded to come. They were - the response was huge! We saved May and we were then able to set about tackling June. We only had one negative response from our mailing. The lady in question said that everyone should stay at home until the disease went away. We didn't reply, but if we had, we would have made the point that if everyone did stay at home then we wouldn't have a home to stay at!

Meanwhile we were being sucked into a culture which was alien to us - that of meetings and political lobbying. Because of the arrival of the crisis, we had just discovered that the Tourism Industry (probably the largest employer in the world) is completely unrepresented in the UK. The scene that we imagined was this. At the end of February MAFF discovers foot & mouth disease and

---

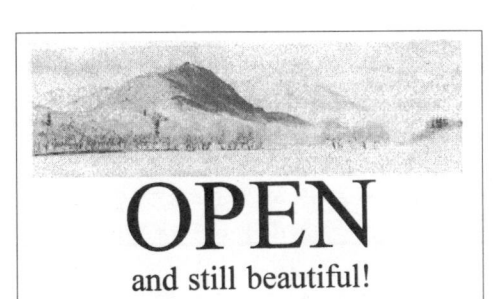

OPEN
and still beautiful!

Contrary to some press reports the Lake District National Park is not closed. Please do come to the Lakes - the views are still magnificent even if you can't climb to the mountain tops or walk on fell footpaths.

We have devised a whole series of walks which enable you to be arrested by the stunning scenery (as opposed to the local constabulary). Four examples are outlined for you overleaf and show you the variety of walks available - some are long & hard, whilst others are for the less energetic. Even seasoned walkers have said how good these walks are, and although they involve walking on minor roads, visitor & vehicle numbers are very low, so movement is free & easy and quiet too!

Almost without exception, all the usual attractions, ornamental gardens, museums etc. are open for visitors. And they and all the small shops, cafes, & businesses will love to see you!

But the warmest welcome of all awaits you here at the Bridge House Hotel in Grasmere - Real Food, Real Fires, Relaxation Guaranteed!

Bridge House Hotel
Church Bridge, Grasmere, Cumbria, LA22 9SN - Tel 015394 35425
www.bridgehousegrasmere.co.uk

brings this to the attention of the UK's 'Senior Management'. Something must be done. So, they blow the cobwebs off the file which says '67 to 68 FMD Outbreak' and read the first few pages. Then they decide to close the countryside. They arrange for everyone in the entire world to get the message 'stay away from Britain's countryside'. And all of a sudden there's a knock at the door. 'Who's that?' they ask. 'It's Tourism, we'd like to know what you want us to do now that you've closed the countryside' comes the reply. 'Who? Tourism? - Never heard of you!'

They've heard of Tourism now, mainly because of Cumbria Crisis Alliance's work, but it remains to be seen whether they're listening or not.

It is now August and the footpaths are open again here in Grasmere. The village is busy with lots of people. Keswick, however, remains a big problem. The footpaths there are not yet open and the main worry is how businesses are to survive the looming winter months.

However, for us, the worst aspect of this continuing crisis is the psychological one. We simply cannot understand what has happened. We see sheep every day. They come into our garden. They enter the school playground where our daughter goes to school, and the children chase them out again. There are sheep on the pavements and roads. Yet humans represent a bio-security threat to them? We cannot get our heads round these fundamental issues. The fact that we have destroyed millions of animals so far. We've polluted our land, our water and our air. We've broadcast the most gruesome pictures of these grotesque measures to the world and, as a result, we've finished people's livelihoods. We cannot understand these things, but we have come to understand a brand new vocabulary - 'bio-security' means walkers dipping their boots at supervised fell access points; we say 'cull' when we mean 'kill' and we burn carcasses on 'pyres' instead of 'fires'. These new words make it sound far more acceptable, don't they? We think our hotel will survive but we don't know about our neighbours in Keswick. We suspect some of them will be taken out in 'contiguous' bankruptcies!

NO ENTRY: Animal Disease Control Precautions

John Collier

John and Anne Collier run Blackdyke Farm Riding Centre at Blackford between Longtown and Carlisle. It is a large riding school with nearly 50 horses employing several members of staff. In the first week of the outbreak alone, they lost £2500, and in the following weeks found their business further diminished; they cancelled all equestrian events and their clients stayed at home, heeding government advice not to venture into the countryside. But the biggest blow of foot and mouth came towards the end of June. This is John's diary from that time.

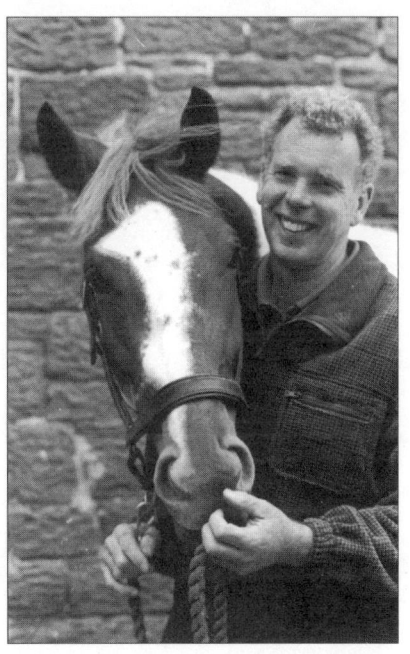

Photo: Expo Life

Friday 22nd June

Four of us are sat around the kitchen table: myself, Anne - my wife, Jayne - the head girl, and Peter, a reporter. It has been a stressful week. Radio Cumbria announced on Monday that DEFRA was going to close all riding schools within 3 km of confirmed cases. This would include us so I have spent all week trying to get some sense from someone: DEFRA, The British Horse Society, David Maclean – and still no joy. Things came to a head yesterday with my calm announcement to the world on BBC Radio Cumbria that if they shut us down we will block the M6 between England and Scotland. This might sound extreme, but we can see no logic in their decision whatsoever. If we were allowed to hold riding lessons last week, why is it any less safe to hold them this week? If farmers are allowed to congregate at DEFRA HQ to pick up licenses for silaging and every other activity on farms, how can we possibly pose any greater threat of spreading foot and mouth than they do?

The police phoned at 10.00 this morning asking my intentions. As usual Anne fielded the call. She assured the policeman that I am serious, even to the point that I have been talking to last year's fuel tax protesters for advice. They want to join in, because they had such a good time last year!

The phone goes non-stop. I ring DEFRA at Rosehill in Carlisle again, and eventually get through. Blunt to the point, I say that if someone doesn't come back to me soon I will come to Rosehill and put a brick through the window. After five days with no reasonable explanations or answers, I'm now starting to understand why people resort to direct action.

We have a funeral to go to at midday: Karl Ebel, our German POW blacksmith. It's a long, sad service. We arrive back in the yard to find two policemen wanting to offer advice about my threatening behaviour. Sudden realisation that DEFRA officials are devoid of any sense of humour! One very nice police lady stays on to make sure that we are OK. We hear that later today DEFRA is going to serve us with a Notice 38 'prohibiting the movement of persons, vehicles and animals' on and off our premises. This means that we can't hold riding lessons, our staple means of income. My temper soars; decide that I will take my battle to the enemy. I drive the horsebox (it's big) down to Rosehill and pull up outside the DEFRA front entrance only to be told 'you can't park here'. 'Just watch this', I say, as I jump out with the keys. I say I won't leave until I can speak to someone and get a doorman who insists on telling me there's no one inside. It's 6.30 p.m. I say I won't leave until I have spoken to a DEFRA official. Twenty minutes later I meet Ray Anderson, DEFRA's Head of Operations in Carlisle – very affable, very reasonable, but no help, so I return home frustrated.

Back home, I ask the police lady (still nice and still here) if she will ask the DEFRA official coming to serve the Notice 38 on us if she'll delay while I get a solicitor. They both agree. It's now 8.40 p.m. and we are all in the kitchen in a stand-off. My dad, aged 83, is staying with us. He walks into the kitchen and collapses over the sink. I manage to get him through to the sitting room and onto the sofa. I ring our local doctor and then decide it looks too serious and phone for an ambulance. I have this vivid picture of Dad being carried out of the kitchen into the ambulance by the doctor and paramedics while this woman from DEFRA decides that now is the ideal time to serve us with our Notice 38.

I tell Dad not to fight my battles. It's quite ironic to think he came to Carlisle for peace and quiet to escape from the race riots in Oldham where he lives!

Arrive home from the hospital at midnight. Fax Tony Blair very politely asking why they are closing us down? Don't sleep.

Saturday 7.15 a.m.
The phone starts. It rings all day: friends, family, supporters, media. Closing the M6 suddenly seems a step closer and the level of support we are getting is fantastic. Anne gets two policemen to accompany her to DEFRA, Rosehill, for 8.30 a.m. to get a statement from Andrew Hayward, Head of Veterinary Operations in Carlisle, to say we are allowed to take riding lessons. It happens, believe it or not, and hey presto, we are open again. Moral of the story: if you want anything done, send a woman. Seethe silently all morning.

Mid afternoon – I go back to DEFRA and let them know that I will not accept their Notice 38 and request a meeting. Not possible they say. No one works at the weekend. Apart from us, of course. And the farmers. And the hoteliers. And everyone else involved in tourism. I phone and phone, again and again.

Sunday 7.30 a.m.
I start phoning again. Want to organise a meeting with DEFRA to get this mess sorted out. No progress. At 10.30 a.m. eventually get someone in the Carlisle office. I tell the lady that I want a meeting. Getting very low on patience by now after nearly a week of trying to resolve this. Tell her that unless I get a meeting I will go on Border TV at lunchtime, explain their policy on leaking cull wagons, and how it doesn't take a genius to work out the spread of the infection along the M6/A66 corridor. Ray Anderson, the boss, comes on the phone and meeting is arranged for 3.00 p.m., my agenda.

Must be a Sunday. No biscuits with the coffee. Explain how we have supported the farmers every bit of the way. How Anne's family are farmers, how our clients and neighbours are farmers. Explain how we tolerate the stench and possible health risks from Hespin Wood, where thousands of slaughtered animals are being tipped just half a mile away from our home and business. Highlight their leaking vehicle policy, and finally show our trump card, a letter from MAFF dated 6th of May saying that we pose no risk to the spread of foot and mouth. The meeting collapses with full apologies.

Monday
We had said that Wednesday was to be the day of the M6 protest. I had liaised with the police. A fax came from DEFRA at lunchtime lifting the Notice 38, pending new risk assessments. Keeping my side of the bargain I stop the demonstration. There are a lot of disappointed people.

P.M. Went to the dentist. Think my dentist is an undercover DEFRA official. He hurt! Gathering of the clans. Sister arrives and we go to see Dad in the Cumberland. Phone calls of support from Alan Coulthard who farms at Justicetown and Margaret Porter at Newtown Farm, up the road. I wonder if they will ever know how much their support meant to us?

Anne speaks to Ray Anderson who tells her that he had been briefed by his media staff that she is a very powerful lady! Think they're referring to 'Tony Blair day', the PM's first visit to Carlisle, when much to my embarrassment she screeched at our illustrious leader and managed to get on all the major news bulletins, the front page of the next day's 'Telegraph', and pretty well every documentary about foot and mouth ever since. At home the children commented that she was shouting at Tony Blair just like she shouted at them. They weren't far wrong either. Except I suspect Tony Blair eats up all his supper like a good boy and goes to bed when he's told. Anne tells Ray Anderson that if things don't get resolved there will most definitely be a protest, and not a half-hearted affair either; she'll go on TV and ask everyone who has a grievance of any sort

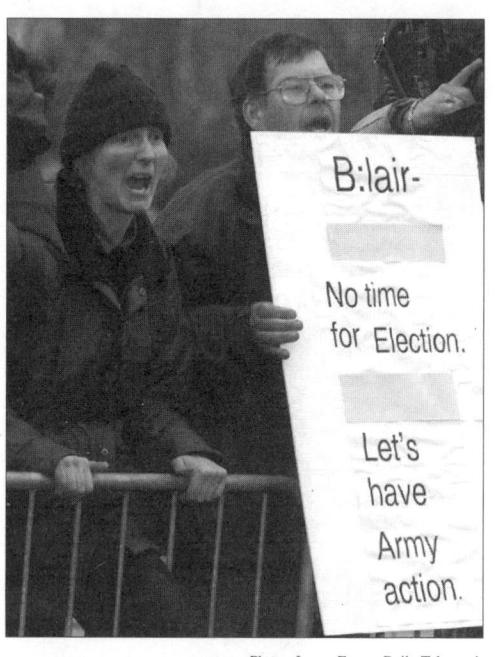

. Photo: James Fraser, Daily Telegraph

with the handling of foot and mouth to come out and show their colours. Border TV come and interview her. It's a good interview and for once she's not wearing that stupid blue woolly hat!

Looking back on all of this a couple of months later, you'll be pleased to hear that Dad got better. I still don't know why they decided to close us down. I feel a bit older and a bit wiser, but I'm left with a bitter taste. My heart goes out to all those poor farmers who have to deal with DEFRA red tape on a daily basis.

Stewart Young

Stewart Young was Leader of Cumbria County Council and Chair of the Cumbria Foot and Mouth Disease Task Force through the early months of the outbreak.

It was Friday 30th March 2001 and I was sitting in the lounge at Carlisle Airport with Carlisle MP Eric Martlew and the County Council's Chief Executive, Louis Victory waiting for Michael Meacher's plane to arrive. It was only the previous week that I had chaired the first meeting of the Cumbria Foot & Mouth Task Force and eight days since the first visit of the Prime Minister to Cumbria. Michael Meacher had been appointed Head of the National Rural Task Force and we were determined to let him see for himself what the situation was like in the worst affected county in the country.

After coffee and a briefing at a nearby hotel, we set off for Longtown. Fires could be seen burning in fields along the side of the road and as we approached the town, there was the unmistakable smell of burning carcasses.

Feelings were running high in Longtown, the epicentre of the outbreak. People were angry and frightened and looking for answers. I knew they would be hard to come by. The Minister met first with the Parish Council and listened while they related their experiences. We then moved into a second meeting with representatives from various businesses in

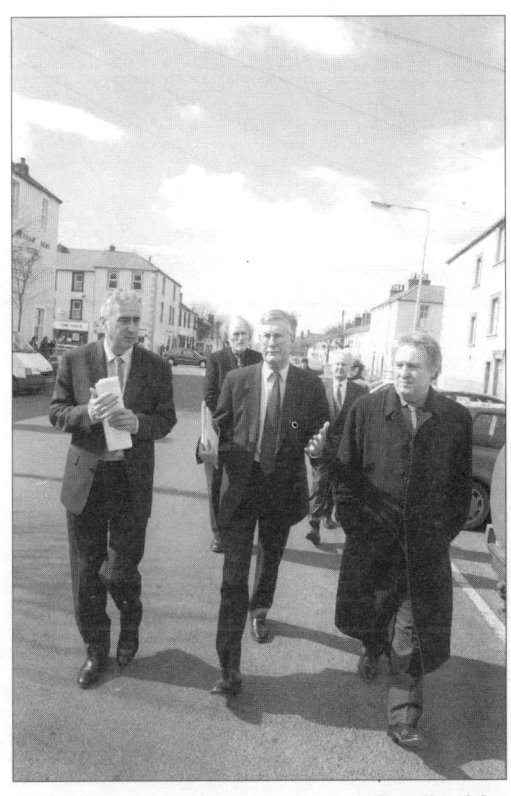

Photo: News & Star

Michael Meacher in Longtown

the town which nearly all depend directly or indirectly on agriculture for their income. When we left the meeting we were faced with a barrage of journalists and film crews, both local and national, anxious to make the lunchtime bulletins. As I watched the obligatory photo opportunity, I wondered what the Minister would make of Longtown and what Longtown would make of the Minister.

We left the town and headed south to Penrith for a private briefing with the other political Group Leaders on the County Council, followed by the Steering Group of the Cumbria Foot & Mouth Task Force representing all the key farming, tourism and business interests in the county. There followed a press conference during which I presented a copy of our Task Force Communiqué, setting out our plea for assistance from Government.

Our next stop was Keswick, where we met representatives from Cumbria Crisis Alliance and a number of businesses in the town. The meeting took place at the Keswick home of the then Member of Parliament for Workington, Dale Campbell-Savours.

Again, this was a very fraught meeting with a number of business representatives explaining how their income had been decimated since footpaths had been closed in the area and visitors had not been able to get access to the fells. It was emphasised that it was not just primary tourism businesses that were affected, but other support services, and that the real difficulties were likely to be over the coming winter, when capital expenditure plans would be deferred and non-vital expenditure cut back. It was remarkable to see, as has been the case throughout the crisis, how tourism and farming interests were supporting each other in recognition of their interdependence. What also came across very strongly was that although businesses in the 'honeypot' areas including towns such as Keswick, had a better chance of survival, those away from the main centres, in the valleys catering exclusively for walkers, were having extreme difficulties.

This was part of the reason for the last visit of the day which was to Whitehaven to meet the local MP, Jack Cunningham, and representatives from some of the businesses in the western valleys, which were, if anything, more deeply affected by the downturn in trade. It also helped to give the Minister an indication of the sheer size of the County and the contrasts between the National Park areas in the centre and the industrialized coastal strip.

At Whitehaven the Minister was again able to hear, first hand, the effect on the local economy, particularly businesses in Wasdale and Eskdale following the unexpected outbreak in the Duddon Valley.

It was by now 6 p.m. and we had to make our way back to Carlisle

Airport and the flight to London. On the way we talked over what we had seen and heard and how we could move things forward. The Minister felt it was important that the National Task Force should hear, first hand what was happening in Cumbria and he invited us to attend their next meeting in London to give a presentation. Immediately following that meeting the Minister announced the first £15 million of Government funding for areas affected by foot & mouth, of which Cumbria was to receive £5 million.

As we made our way towards Carlisle, the Minister reminisced about a holiday he had spent in the area many years before, during which time he had played a game of tennis on a municipal court in Aspatria which he claimed was the best such tennis court he had ever played on. I wonder what became of it?

We arrived at Carlisle Airport on schedule. I had to be in London myself that evening and as my own travel arrangements had been disrupted due to the Ministerial visit, I hitched a lift. As we landed at RAF Northolt after a 45-minute flight I decided that this was a preferable way to travel than the West Coast main line. This was to prove all too accurate when my return journey to Carlisle two days later took 8 hours!

Looking back on the day's events, I felt we had been able to get across some strong messages to Government about the situation in Cumbria and that in Michael Meacher, we had a strong ally. However, I knew that the real battle would be with the Treasury but that was for another day.

NO ENTRY: Animal Disease Control Precautions

Andrew Beeforth

This is the story of the Cumbria Community Recovery Fund, an initiative of the Cumbria Community Foundation, told by the Foundation's Director, Andrew Beeforth. All profits from the sales of this book will go to support the work of the Recovery Fund.

On the 28th February 2001 I met with a number of Trustees to review the first year of the Foundation and to plan for the future. Little did we know what effect the foot and mouth outbreak would have on Cumbria and the Community Foundation. A few days later the number of cases of foot and mouth nationally, and particularly in Cumbria began to spiral out of control. As foot and mouth disease and its effects grew it became clear that the Foundation might be able to help. As the only Charitable Trust dedicated to Cumbria it was possible that we could try and raise significant sums of money.

I was not confident that we could achieve this. No UK Community Foundation had ever launched an appeal like this before. We were very new and I wasn't sure whether it was fair to place so much work on a small and already busy team of staff and volunteers. Although we were confident of our ability to make good use of any monies raised we did not want to let people down by raising expectations which could not be met. We were aware that if an appeal were to be launched that we should seek to raise enough money to make a difference. After a short discussion with my chairman we proposed a £1.2m target.

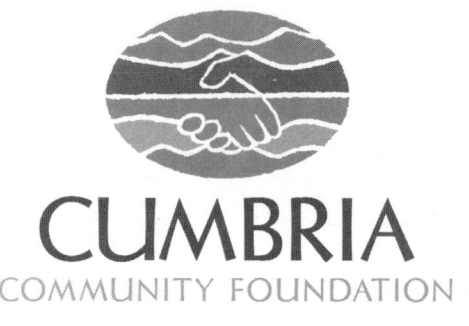

I was heartened by the early support of the Kendal based Francis C Scott Charitable Trust, whose Trustees agreed a donation of £50,000 to the Fund. Along with £20,000 of the Foundation's own money and the endorsement of the County Foot and Mouth Task Force it was all systems go......and on 3rd April 2001, Sir Chris Bonington launched the Cumbria Community Recovery Fund on behalf of the Community Foundation.

The following weeks saw many new volunteers, a County Council secondee and Territorial Army soldiers introduced to the Foundation. My chairman dedicated many hours to the preparation of applications to charitable trusts, filling in as receptionist and envelope stuffer when my PA broke her toe!

Over 60,000 appeal leaflets and posters were distributed in the early weeks of the appeal. The response was overwhelming, to date the Fund has received over 1200 individual donations. At one stage a full time volunteer was dedicated to recording and banking cheques. Groups from all over Cumbria ran fund-raising events, serving coffee, holding concerts and rattling tins for the Fund. Prince Charles provided his endorsement to the Fund. Jancis Robinson, one of Cumbria's most acclaimed celebrities, gave a special wine tasting which raised £15,000.

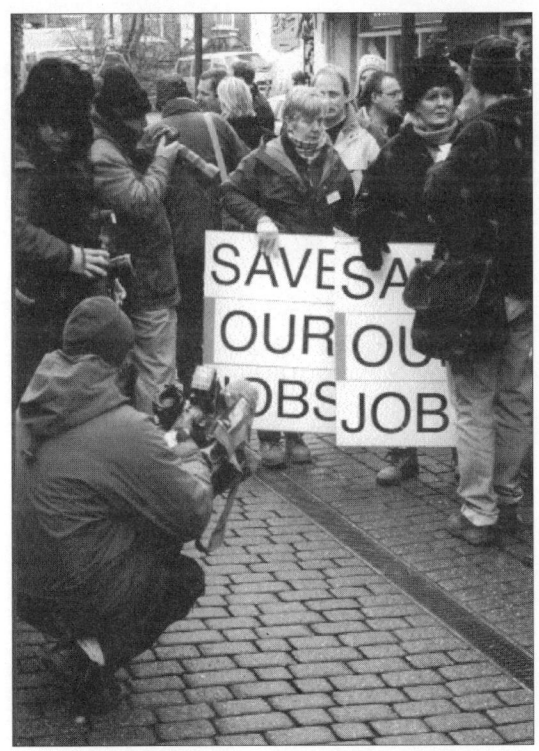

Photo: Keith James, Keswick Reminder
Cumbria Crisis Alliance campaigns for support for businesses in Keswick

The management of the Fund has been a deeply emotional experience for everyone involved. Each day our staff and volunteers have spoken to people who are experiencing the potential loss of their livelihoods. Staff and volunteers responded extraordinarily to the challenge. A colleague from the California Community Foundation (who are donors to the Fund) compared our experience to their own response to earthquakes. At times people were working in quite challenging conditions. On one occasion 12 people were working in two small offices, with the chairman dealing with correspondence cross legged in the middle of the floor using a suitcase as a desk!

The warmth and generosity of donors has been a feature of the Fund. It has provided a tangible way for people to express their sympathy. Many people have been deeply moved by what has happened and have expressed grief for Cumbria and the Lake District.

'Dear Sir,
Having seen your Appeal in the Church Times (which I get surface mail) I am enclosing a cheque for £50. I have fond memories of the Lake District as I was evacuated during the war to Rydal Hall. I do hope the area and indeed the whole of the UK will recover from the devastation of foot and mouth.'

Lesmurdie, Western Australia

'For over 20 years I've lived and worked as a GP in old mining communities. I know it is not exactly the same, but I have seen and heard what happens to people in communities when employment is wiped out of an area – I hope your fund helps people recover and start again.'

Houghton Le Spring, Tyne and Wear.

'This is the sum of a collection made at the Christening of our daughter's baby in Switzerland.'

Rosley, Wigton.

'Enclosed is a donation for £12 to the Recovery Fund. This is from my mother-in-law, who is 91 and currently in hospital. She won the £12 in the ward sweepstake on the Grand National and was most insistent that it should be sent to you to help the farmers.'

Lincoln

'Please find enclosed a cheque for £10 for the Farmers of Cumbria. My heart goes out to them all. Although I now live in Lancashire I was brought up on the West side of Derwentwater. Please save the Herdwick sheep – the only ones I used to see in that area.'

Preston

At the time of writing this, £1.3m has been raised of which £300,000 had been distributed by early August with 97 community groups and 180 individual hardship cases supported. Groups funded have included support organisations such as CAB and Samaritans which have increased their services to help people affected by the crisis and grants to groups looking to help with the re-building process including farm diversification and training projects.

One beneficiary from the Cumbria Community Recovery Fund had explained 'the grant will help pay the bills, but more importantly has helped boost our confidence that we will be able to bring our farming enterprise back from the edge, and survive'.

As coverage of foot and mouth disease diminishes from the national press I am aware that the work of the Foundation is far from over. The Fund has a new appeal target (£1.8m). The Foundation also continues to seek support for the development of its endowment fund, which will provide the resources required for long term grant making to benefit communities in Cumbria.

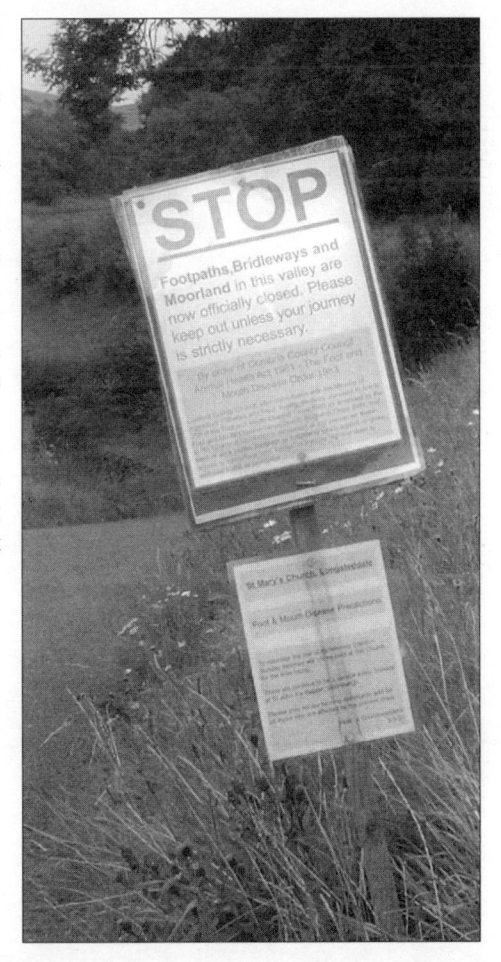

Valerie Edmondson

Valerie Edmondson is a National Park Ranger covering an area around Keswick. She is also a farmer. Her job found her dealing with worried farmers desperate to keep the virus away from their stock as well as those in the tourist industry who were equally desperate to see fell paths reopened to support their ailing businesses. This is her personal recollection of the foot and mouth outbreak and does not necessarily reflect the views of the Lake District National Park Authority.

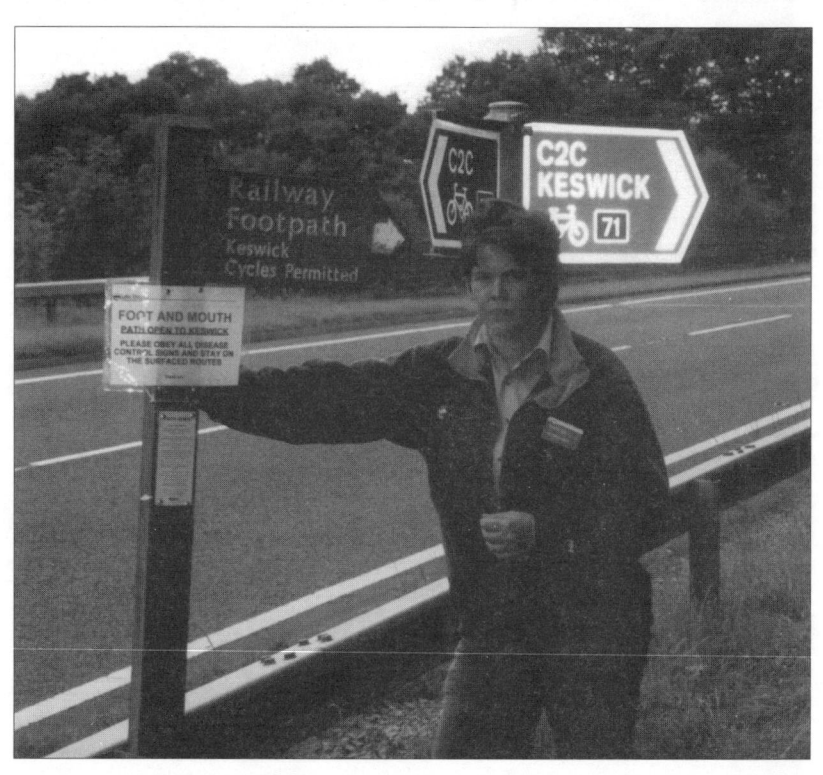

Being born and bred on a hill farm in the Lake District and after working on local farms, I landed my job as a Lake District National Park Authority Ranger in 1989. Although well aware that in many people's eyes I had the perfect job, there was still something missing – the opportunity to work amongst livestock. A couple of years later and following consultation with my employers, my brother and I took on the tenancy of a small sheep and beef farm in the Borrowdale Valley. My days off and most of my holidays are spent on the farm working with our sheep and cattle. It provides an excellent contrast to my work as a National Park Authority Ranger.

In February of this year my whole world was turned on its head following reports of foot and mouth in the county. All footpaths and bridleways in the area were closed. Firstly a voluntary ban was imposed and then the County Council enforced official closures of all rights of way in the area. National Park Authority Rangers, Estate staff, Voluntary Wardens and National Trust staff were involved in the massive signing exercise. Dozens of desperate farmers were ringing the office pleading for signs to keep people off their land until this dreadful disease had gone away. I became involved with National Trust Wardens, local farmers and County Highways officers organising disinfectant mats across roads leading into valleys such as Newlands and Borrowdale. Our Voluntary Wardens were available at weekends to advise the few visitors to the area of the restrictions in place.

The national papers and news were all about the dreadful plague which was sweeping the county. As time went on I began to recognise the odd name of infected farms from old auction catalogues, then I knew the farmers themselves and things were really serious. Hearing of close friends having all their stock slaughtered and dumped under their noses for weeks to rot really did shake me, like a bereavement, and I felt the very least I could do was to send sympathy cards to express my condolences. The feeling of loss must have been felt by many others as it wasn't long before the local papers were full of thanks for sympathy from victims of the foot and mouth crisis.

Meanwhile, back at work, the enquiries kept coming. People with guest houses wondering how long the paths would remain closed, outdoor recreation centres desperate for somewhere to run their training sessions, together with the general public ringing to find out what was open if they should choose to visit the area.

The 3km voluntary cull introduced in April then brought the whole thing home. We had our old faithful Blue Faced Leicester tups off wintering on a farm near Abbeytown, along with 75 other breeding tups from the Borrowdale valley. Some were the highest quality Herdwick tups you can get. The phone rang and I was suddenly being asked to 'give up' our tups in a voluntary cull. I think not! As long as this cull is voluntary we will not give our tups up for slaughter. One tup is nine years old and has become part of the family. He has given a lifetime of good service and I wasn't ready to condemn him to death, especially in a 'voluntary' cull.

Over the next few days the calls continued and my heels dug in deeper. A friend with Herdwick tups wintering on the same farm was having the same hassle and was desperately trying to get a scheme together to at least save some semen from the tups which were by now on death row. Foot and mouth was then confirmed on the farm and all the tups were culled. The last sighting we had of our tups was on the television one evening when Border Television showed a feature on the scheme to take semen from Herdwick tups to save the breed. It was very sad to see our tups race across the screen, they looked so healthy and now they were all dead. Our first and second prize Swaledale gimmer hoggs, with a lifetime ahead of them went the same way – they were all stranded on a farm near Skelton.

Every farmer in the area had similar tales of death: some lost hoggs, shearlings and ewes, leaving a gap in their flock which can never be filled. With the slaughtered sheep went their hefting instinct, a unique ability to stay on a certain area of fell without straying, despite there being no fences. It is therefore not an option for fell farmers to 'top up' with brought in sheep.

As time went on it soon became clear that closing all rights of way down for a couple of months until the disease went away was not the answer. The disease was obviously here to stay, for this year at least. On the one hand the best solution is for everyone to stay away from the area to avoid the spread of the disease. On the other, people were needed to visit and spend money on accommodation and in shops generally, to keep a dying tourism industry trade alive.

Rangers were busy risk-assessing paths, properties and other access areas in an attempt to open up some safe places for people to go. I began to risk-assess the Keswick to Threlkeld Railway footpath, a very popular route open for walkers, cyclists and wheelchair users. Past surveys had revealed over 500 users in any one day. Parish Councils were supportive of the proposal to open the route, local caravan sites and pubs were also keen, and even the adjacent farmers and landowners understood the plight of the tourism trade and supported the opening with a few precautionary measures in place. Then we had a confirmed case just east of Keswick which threw most of the Railway Footpath into a 3km protection zone. We were back to square one.

By now pressure from the tourism trade

STOP!
FOOT & MOUTH DISEASE

It is now unlawful to use this path (possible penalty £5,000)

All footpaths and bridleways across fells, other farmland and through woodland are now closed to public use. Foot and Mouth is a contagious disease which threatens the way of life of everyone in rural communities.

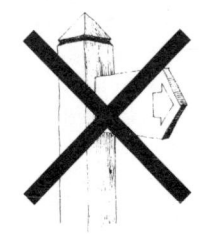

For further information, please telephone 0845 6014068

was really building. The whole area was quiet, people were staying away and we needed something to bring them back. Some stayed away thinking it the right and proper thing to do, some were picking up confused messages and thought they were being told to stay away, and some did come and had an enjoyable stay, but others were annoyed that they had been brought here under false pretences, led to believe that the National Park was open for business even though most of the rights of way remained closed.

Another popular path on the outskirts of Keswick and outside the new 3km zone was felt to be a suitable route which could be worth pursuing. The farmer in question was very aware of the desperate situation regarding tourism in the area, but felt that it was a little too early to be opening paths through his livestock. With bank holiday approaching and funds available he agreed to erect over 300m of temporary buffer zone fencing to keep the public and his cattle separated. The path was safely opened ready for the May bank holiday. A steady stream of people used the path for six days until a new case of foot and mouth was confirmed at Keswick throwing a 3km protection zone around that path too. DEFRA ordered its immediate closure.

After three months and with a tourism industry now on its knees, it was felt that the only thing to bring back visitors was to reopen some of the high fells. 'Consultation' meetings were arranged to allow farmers and landowners to comment. Many were frightened and annoyed by the proposals to allow all and sundry back on the fells amongst the few sheep that until now had managed to escape being culled. Assurances were given that the risks were minimal and visitors would access the fells via designated, manned disinfectant points with no access for dogs. Very reluctantly the farmers accepted the idea and June 9th dawned. Farmers' fears were fuelled when it emerged that the foot dips at each site were merely detergent. The disinfectant did not arrive until the following day.

Although most people were behaving responsibly, Rangers were fielding calls from people reporting dogs on the fells, people straying from the designated access points and accessing or leaving the fells via closed paths without disinfecting. Not to mention the couple camping on the field at Castlerigg Stone Circle where infected sheep had been slaughtered just weeks before!

Visitor numbers did increase with the news that the Lake District fells had reopened, but with the school holidays approaching it was felt that more low-level paths should open throughout the country. However, it was recognised that Cumbria, being the worst hit county in terms of confirmed cases, should be an exemption to the proposed blanket lifting of the ban on use of rights of way. A map was prepared which highlighted areas away from any previous infection where it was felt the paths could open safely. Letters were sent out by Cumbria County Council and DEFRA informing farmers of the latest proposals. Farmers had a few weeks to appeal against any particular paths on their farms opening if they led the public into areas where stock congregated, such as sheep pens and cattle yards.

This was the hardest time of all for me personally. Any farmers who were not National Trust or United Utilities tenants had to appeal via their local Ranger to discuss the new access proposals. Many hadn't left their holdings for months and were desperately concerned that the general public would soon be trailing over their land, this time without being disinfected!

The timing couldn't have been worse. The farmers had just received a video from DEFRA promoting strict bio-security followed a few days later by a letter telling them that the paths across their land would be reopening. The phones started ringing and didn't stop for a week. Farmers were annoyed, depressed and worried and each had their own horrible story to tell. Everyone I dealt with was frustrated, most had lost large quantities of stock in the voluntary, contiguous or 3km culls. Others were desperately trying to sort out movement licences to get starving stock moved onto fresh pastures or bulls in with cows. One farmer had been making hay only to find he was not allowed to deliver it to his barn. It was left to waste in the rain.

According to DEFRA risk assessment guidelines the risk posed by walkers is minimal, so only a handful of paths remained closed in the designated access areas and a few diversions were set up around sheep pens etc. On August 1st fell access points were removed and many low-level paths were reopened. Later in August the 3km restrictions were lifted in the Keswick area. All stock had been blood tested and results were negative. A ray of hope?

My greatest fear now is that the disease may return to an area that is slowly returning to some normality. The time of year is fast approaching when all farmers would normally sell their lambs and suckled calves, but everything is so uncertain this year and no one knows what lies ahead for the tourism sector. A black cloud still hangs over the area and very few conversations end without a mention of foot and mouth in some shape or form.

This year is the 50th anniversary of the Lake District National Park. I feel that the area will look very different in the next 50 years due to this terrible foot and mouth epidemic of 2001.

Throughout the last six months I have felt 'stuck in the middle', trying to support a desperate tourism trade whilst attempting to support everything which may discourage the spread of the virus. I have spoken on the phone to farmer's wives in tears and then received calls from irate guest house owners accusing me of losing them trade by keeping the paths closed. It has been a really trying time and I sincerely hope that the worst is over and that I never experience foot and mouth ever again.

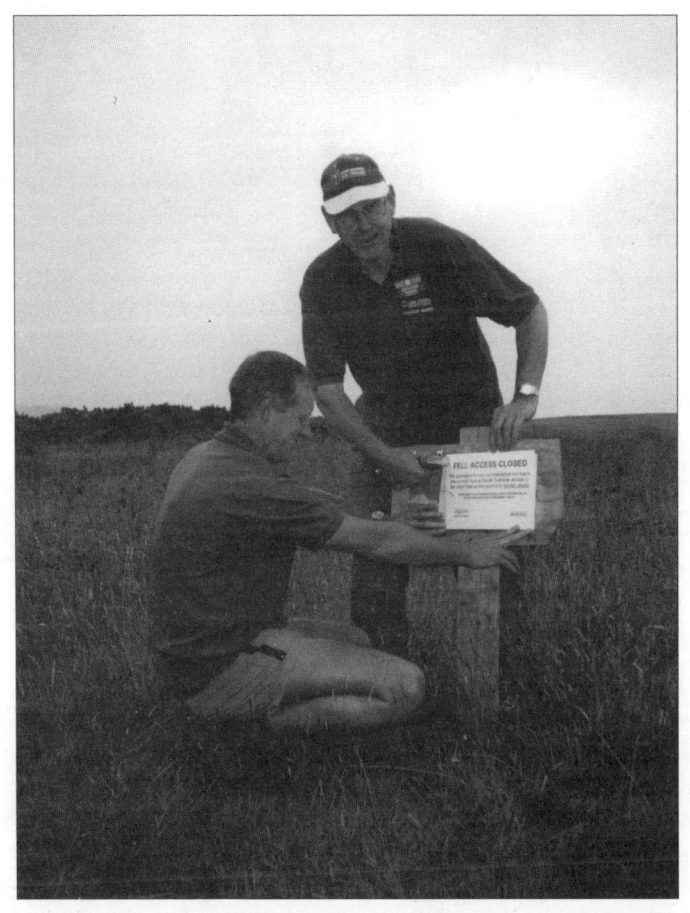

Ranger Colin Eastham and voluntary Ranger Dennis Forrest putting up 'Fell Access Closed' signs.

Oliver Maurice

Oliver Maurice is the Director of the National Trust for the North West Region. The Trust owns nearly 100 hill farms and a fifth of the total Herdwick population. Many of its non-farming tenants rely on a constant stream of tourists throughout the summer months to keep their businesses ticking over.

The year 2000 will be remembered not only for the celebrations surrounding the start of a new millennium but also for the appallingly wet autumn coupled with the petrol crisis. The effect of this on visitor numbers to the Lake District was disastrous for many tourism-related businesses. The light at the end of the tunnel however was that advanced bookings for the coming year were well up on 2000 for many of those businesses and the Cumbria Tourist Board was forecasting a very good year.

Within the National Trust's Regional Office at Grasmere there was a sense of optimism that 2001 might prove a turning point from the previous 2 or 3 years of falling visitor numbers to our properties. All too early in the year our hopes were dashed.

The news of the first outbreak of foot and mouth in Essex on the 20th February rang few alarm bells at the time as it seemed so far away. Two days later when it was traced back to a farm at Heddon-on-the-Wall I became concerned. When Longtown Auction Mart became the focus of attention it was time to take action.

A colleague came in to my office and said, 'I think we should take this seriously' and I agreed.

From that day in March until the beginning of August all previously planned work went by the board and my life became totally focused on preventing the spread of the disease.

Perhaps the blackest day of all for me was a Saturday in March when I received a telephone call at home from a vet at Blackhall Farm in the Duddon.

'Mr Maurice' he said, 'your tenant suggested I ring to let you know that five minutes ago I diagnosed foot and mouth disease in his cattle.' My heart sank. I knew then that could be the death knell for large numbers of Herdwick sheep in the vicinity and conceivably throughout the fells. The National Trust owns and protects approximately one quarter of the Lake District National Park including 91 hill farms. Most of them are in the western and central fells and are contiguous one with another.

The Trust also owns approximately one fifth of the total population of

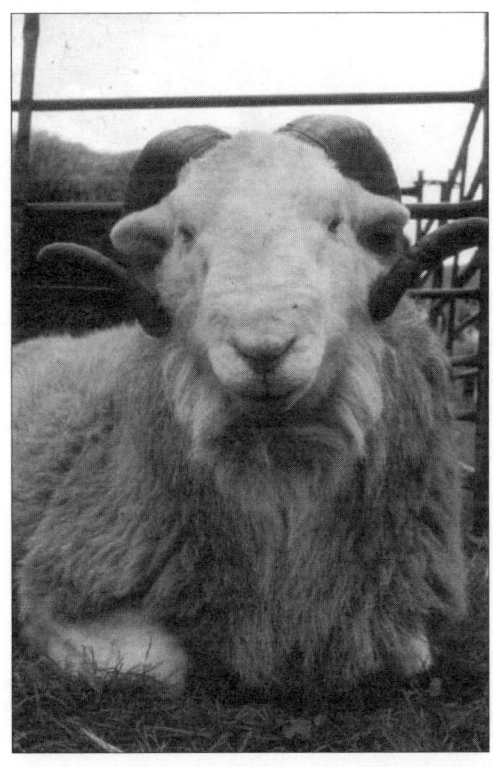

The hardy and distinctive Herdwick sheep (Photo: National Trust)

Herdwicks (21,000) which it lets to its tenants as the 'landlord's flock'. Our 91 tenants between them own a further 30,000 or so. Between us half the population of this indigenous breed lives on Trust land. These were the statistics before the outbreak.

The vet told me that all the animals on Blackhall Farm and on the neighbouring Cockley Beck farm would have to be slaughtered. I remember feeling a sense of utter despair and helplessness as an initial reaction. I then went into overdrive and spent most of the rest of the weekend on the telephone to colleagues, to the two tenants to express my deepest sympathies and planning for an emergency meeting on the Monday.

At the time there were differing views as to the cause. The favoured view was that it had been transmitted by wind from the Penrith area but car tyres, walkers and feed lorries all came into the reckoning. Whether we will ever know is open to question.

Nevertheless my instinct told me that I needed to enlist the help of the Police to get all roads to the Duddon closed to visitors and bio-security measures put in place. The Police at Headquarters at Penrith were entirely sympathetic and telephoned me on the Sunday to say that manned roadblocks were in place in Eskdale, Ulpha and at the bottom of Wrynose in Little Langdale. Three days later they telephoned me again to say they were not legally empowered to man the roadblocks and had withdrawn their staff. Nevertheless the signs and disinfectant remained in place and our own staff did what they could to persuade visitors not to use the roads.

The support we had from BBC Radio Cumbria both then and throughout

Photo: National Trust

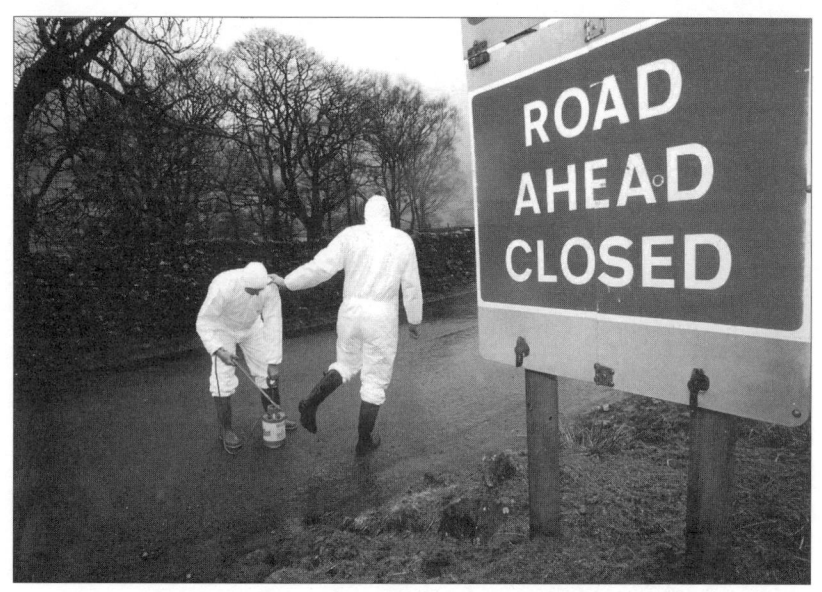

Many roads were temporarily closed as disposal teams went about their work

the crisis was for me one of the plus points. The haunting jingle preceding the voice of Anne Hopper is indelibly cast in my mind and 7.55 a.m. became essential listening each morning when I always tended to fear the worst and learn that yet more National Trust farms had gone down.

In fact it was two weeks before the disease struck another National Trust farm, this time Hazel Head, on Birker Moor, taking three other farms including another Trust farm with it. Again the news broke, this time on a Friday evening and another weekend was spent on the telephone!

Press activity surrounding these outbreaks knew no bounds and I found myself giving interminable interviews to all and sundry. Perhaps the most surprising was the BBC World Service who woke me at 6.30 a.m. one morning wanting to do a live telephone interview ten minutes later!

Throughout the crisis and particularly in the later stages when the footpaths remained closed but the messages were that walkers posed a minimal risk to the spread of the disease, striking a balance between the needs of the farming fraternity and that of the tourist industry became increasingly difficult. Many of our farm tenants were not only suffering through the loss of away wintered livestock caught up in culls elsewhere in Cumbria, and movement restrictions, but also through loss of tourist trade having diversified into B&B, campsites, tea rooms etc. Many of our business tenants were suffering too.

As the disease spread and the hardship increased across the board so the antipathy between tourism and related businesses and the farmers began to intensify. The month of July was the hardest in this respect when I began to receive vitriolic letters laying the blame on me and the Trust for closing everything down.

At the outset of the disease I was an advocate for vaccination of the Herdwicks and I still am today. The argument that it will ruin the export trade cuts little ice with me. I am a firm believer in local markets and adding value to produce through branding, given the necessary quality assurance and traceability; a further benefit is that local markets cut down the 'food miles', the huge distances that live and dead stock are transported before sale. This must be the way forward.

With hindsight, had the Government approved the vaccination of rare and threatened species from the outset, access restrictions on the fells could have been lifted much sooner than they were and many farmers and small businesses would not have suffered the hardship they have.

As a member of the Cumbria Task Force Planning Group I have sensed in recent weeks a strong partnership building up between all those around the table and a huge willingness to move Cumbria out of the doldrums caused by this dreadful disease.

My own organisation is in a strong position to play its part through its ability, as a significant landowner, to put into practice many of the pilot projects stemming from the proposed regeneration and the Trust's own 'Vision for the Lake District after Foot and Mouth'.

NO ENTRY: Animal Disease Control Precautions

Russell Bowman

Russell Bowman farms at Garthfolds Farm, Lazonby. He and his family have a hundred dairy cattle, a small beef herd and gave up 1000 sheep to the voluntary cull. Throughout the crisis he recorded his thoughts in an audio diary that was broadcast on the Richard Nankivell Programme on BBC Radio Cumbria.

Opportunity knocked at my door in the shape of foot and mouth. While other people are content to achieve fame and notoriety by warbling their favourite song on prime time ITV, I had to make do with an audio diary of the various goings-on at Garthfolds. This did have the advantage though of me being able to enjoy my fifteen minutes of fame without anyone having to see my face! As my fiancé said, I have got the perfect face for radio!

A producer from Radio Cumbria, Richard Moss, got in touch with me and asked if I would be willing to record a diary for weekly broadcast. To be honest I have always had an inkling towards doing something like that but I never thought that my chance would come along, and it was a shame that my chance did come along because of the foot and mouth virus. However I have often thought that I could do better than other people who comment on agriculture so here was the chance to see if my overinflated view of myself matched up to reality – Judge for yourself!

The diary itself was recorded on a portable minidisc recorder that Richard delivered before milking time one afternoon. We didn't get off to a good start because we arranged to meet at our next door farm, Craggnook, on the side of the main road and unfortunately Richard got his directions muddled and sped right past me. As we hadn't met previously I had no idea where he was until he realised his mistake and eventually found me. He explained how the recorder worked and to this day we have never met again. Every Wednesday after that I put the previous week's minidisc in the box at the end of our lane which Richard collected and he generally left a spare. I soon began to dread looking in the box on Wednesday night just in case there was no blank disc – that would have meant the end of my contract!

As soon as the first instalment of my diary was broadcast the phone rang. It was a friend to say how much they had enjoyed listening. I can honestly say that the response was amazing and over the six week run of the diary we received around thirty calls, some from locals to say that they had really enjoyed listening and some from complete strangers, one or two of whom were quite emotional after listening to my account of the sheep being taken away to Great Orton. I must admit that not all correspondence was positive, with one person writing to say how disgusted she was with me for allowing our sheep to go to the cull in the first place. Apparently I had said that one reason for letting them go was because I didn't want to go through the cleaning and disinfecting procedure if we had got foot and mouth. Upon listening to the repeat play of the diary I realised that I had, in fact, said that. It made me realise how careful you have to be when you put your thoughts into the public domain. My only defence for this slip was the fact that I generally did my recording after a 16 or 18 hour day.

During the recording of my diary I included some humour, as foot and mouth caused so much unhappiness I thought a few lighter moments would not go amiss. Luckily nearly everyone who listened thought that something along the way was funny and most people found the story about the roller quite amusing. For those who didn't catch it on the radio, this was the story of some daft idiot who left our roller out in a field over winter. As many of you involved in farming will know rollers are often filled with water. If you leave them outside during these cold Cumbrian winters they tend to freeze and burst, a bit like water pipes that haven't been lagged. Well, as I say, some idiot on our farm left ours out through all the worst frosts of the winter and I discovered this while up to my ears with disinfectant, form-filling and foot and mouth scares. It was one of those days, and if I ever get my hands on the bloke that left it outside! (Now who could that have possibly been? Ed.)

The most memorable occasion that has occurred since I became a Radio Cumbria star was the meeting I attended at Newton Rigg College. Along with other young rural people I was asked to attend a meeting in order to put the young person's view of the future of the countryside to the Government Minister Alun Michael. We had our lunch in the college cafeteria and I was just leaving when a lady ran over and asked if I was Russell Bowman. I replied that I was and the lady asked me if I would go and meet one of the staff working in the kitchen. After a few minutes another lady came dashing out and straight away gave me a big hug and a kiss! She said that she always listened to my diary and always looked forward to the next instalment. The worst part was that I have forgotten the lady's name but she certainly made my day. It is nice to know that I have at least one fan!

One last humorous tale occurred last week and almost on my doorstep. A near neighbour applied for and received a license to move sheep from fields near his home back to the main farm to be dipped. His sheep had previously been blood-tested and had been negative. As my neighbour had left the field with the sheep in his cattle trailer, the DEFRA man shouted at him to wait a minute while he shut the gate and then disinfected before getting into his car. The farm in question is about six miles away and along a route that twists and turns through various villages and all along minor roads – not very good to find if you do not know the area. Whether the farmer did not hear him or whether he was getting tired of the DEFRA man we will never know but he sped off. The DEFRA man in his panic shut the gate but somehow managed to drop his mobile phone in the bucket of disinfected water! By the time DEFRA man had got sorted out and in the car our hero was long gone and had not left directions to the farm. The reason I knew what had happened was that DEFRA man pulled in at the junction above our farm to consult his map. I pulled up at the junction to let a car past and he jumped out to ask directions. Apparently by the time DEFRA man arrived at the farm my neighbour had done the job and was loading up ready to come back with his sheep.

I am told my audio diary will resume in the autumn when hopefully there will be more good news to report than there has been of late.

We tried to get hold of a photo of Russell so readers could judge for themselves whether he has indeed got the perfect face for radio, as suggested by his fiancé (now wife), but he was somewhat reluctant to supply one. Why might that be? Last time we spoke to him he was busy capitalising on his new found fame being interviewed by his childhood hero John Craven for BBC1's 'Countryfile' programme. (Ed.)

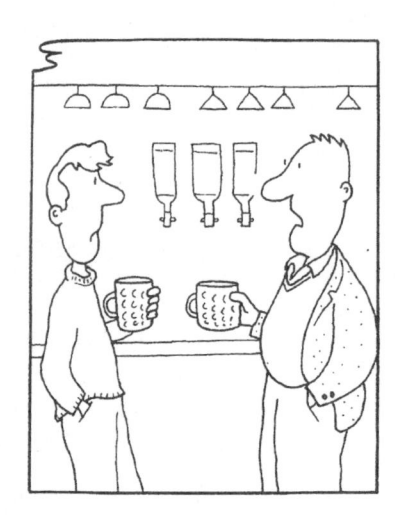

"I work in crisis management - I'm a farmer."

Allan Miller

Allan Miller is a freelance computer programmer who was born in Threlkeld and now lives near Kendal. He spends much of his free time enjoying the Cumbrian hills, fell running, walking and climbing. He is a member of Kendal Amateur Athletic Club's championship winning veterans fell running team.

The Seven Billion Pound Bucket of Swill.

Preparations were well under way for the new fell running season when the news came through - 'Foot and Mouth found at an abattoir in Essex'. Still fat from Christmas, I'd started to do a few Winter League races to build up some fitness and fight the flab. By the weekend, the countryside was closed. Clunk. Just like that. 'Rights' of way turned out to be very fragile rights indeed. The hills were bathed in sunshine and snow, but a trip up to Kirkstone saw the car park shut, and just a few people chucking desultory snowballs.

Even now, six months on, though most of Britain's countryside is 'open for business', and there is no evidence that walkers pose any threat, the paths in my area remain firmly shut. A five thousand pound fine just for running along the canal, so, needs must, I turned into a road runner. It's just not the same though - there's no incentive to go out in the wind and the rain to fight with cars on tarmac, and with no races to aim for. Things went from bad to worse. I ballooned, so the only races of the spring, four times round Kendal Castle, saw me flagging from the off, and beaten by even fatter contenders than myself.

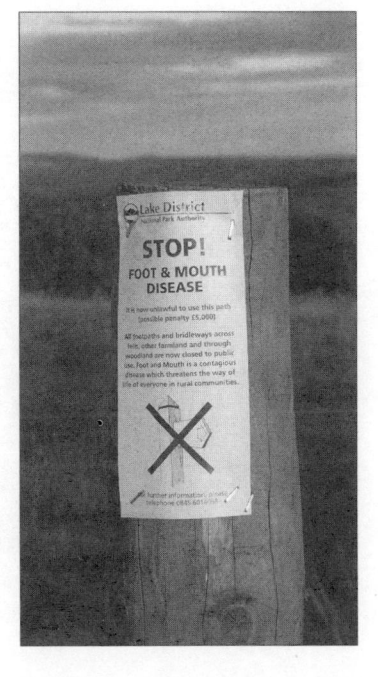

Scotland proved my salvation - they could afford to have a more relaxed policy than England and Wales, having been spared the worst of the disease, so I made regular trips along the A74. These brought home the full horror of the disease control measures, as from Shap to Moffat, not an animal remained. At dusk, smoke rose from a dozen pyres, the fires glowing red against the darkening sky, and the choking stench putting the punters off their burgers at Southwaite Services.

Once in the north, though, I could once again feel turf underfoot, and legitimately leave the roads behind to head into the hills. I followed spring north but, back in the Lakes, the lovely May weather was tarnished by the ongoing ban, and runs round the Lakeland roads met with ample evidence that, even on tarmac, I was not welcome. I sought out the steeper roads, for hill-training - up the Struggle from Ambleside, then back down the Kirkstone Road; over Blea Tarn from Great to Little Langdale; over Red Bank and White Moss; poor substitutes for the real thing but, lacking any real traffic, much better than nothing.

Finally, common sense prevailed, and cautious openings commenced, enabling limited family picnics, off-road runs and climbing. Progress was slow, decisions often illogical, and opinions on opening conflicted even among the experts. It is frightening how readily the countryside can be closed, and liberties we take for granted removed overnight, and yet how painfully slowly it reopens.

So at last, we had the first Lakeland fell race of the year, in Borrowdale in August, on an unmodified course despite recent restrictions at Seathwaite. A flash in the pan, perhaps, because no one has yet followed suit, but a splendid great-to-be-back atmosphere and a reminder of the good old days. Even the Duke of Edinburgh turned up to show his support. And me? Well, I finished, but my running shoes - weakened, I am convinced, by repeated dippings in acid disinfectants - disintegrated a quarter of the way round!

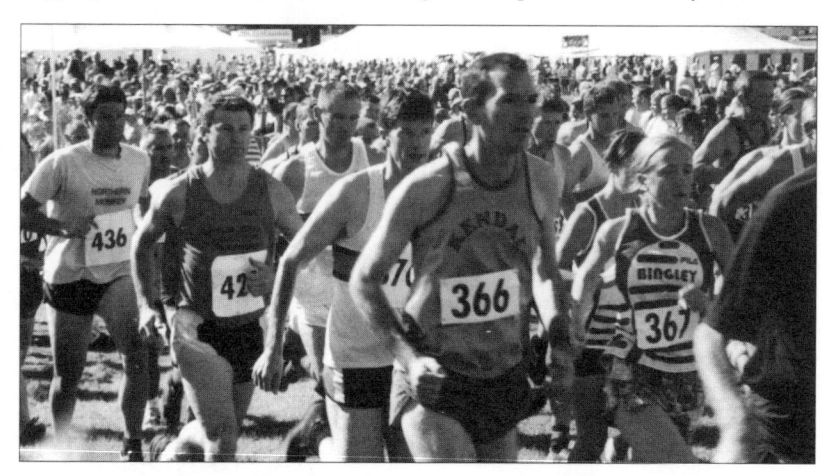

Fell runners flex those muscles at last.
The Senior Guides Race at Grasmere Sports, 2001

Anne Gallagher

Anne Gallagher lives in Hawkshead and runs The Minstrels' Gallery Tea Rooms and a holiday cottage business. She was one of the organisers of Hawkshead Village Fair, a special event planned to pull some much needed tourists into the village.

Wednesday 15th August.
Exactly one week to go before the 'big day'. Gin no longer having the 'oh, everything will be fine' effect. May have to try something stronger. How exactly did I get here, poised somewhere between great expectation and sickening dread? It all seemed a good idea at the time, sitting in the King's Arms, Hawkshead, with a few other locals wondering why, in the middle of May, we were the only people in the pub. Of course I should have realised we were in for a rough time when back in March some American visitors who stay in one of our cottages every year, rang to offer me a food parcel! According to CNN the poor folks in 'Beatrix Potter Land' were all housebound and starving. Hawkshead is a real honeypot. It acts like a magnet to those in search of a typical Lakeland village. However thanks to foot and mouth our village was totally uncontaminated by tourism. Shame really, when most villagers depend on the tourist industry to keep body and soul together.

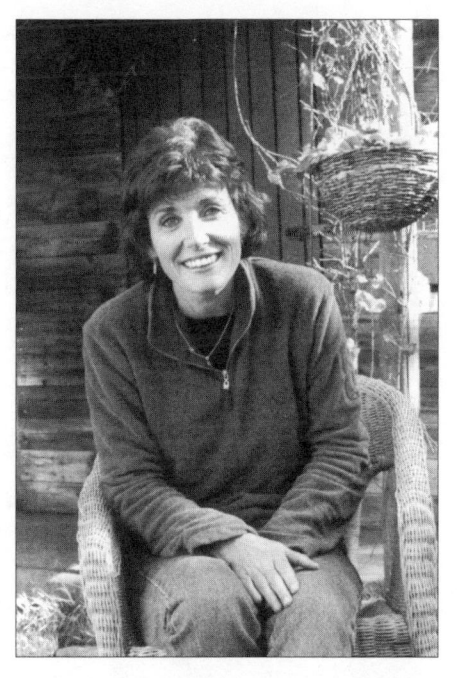

As I remember it, it had become clear that Hawkshead's annual country show was going to be cancelled and that left everyone feeling totally fed up. Almost without exception local people plan a day off on Hawkshead Show Day. It's a chance for our children to prepare artwork and displays for the home craft competitions, for farmers to show off the best of their livestock and for us all to enjoy the many delights in the refreshment tent. We now had to face up to the fact that we would feel the effects of foot and mouth right throughout the summer and beyond. 'We have to do something that will attract people to this village, something big, loud and entertaining', said Ed

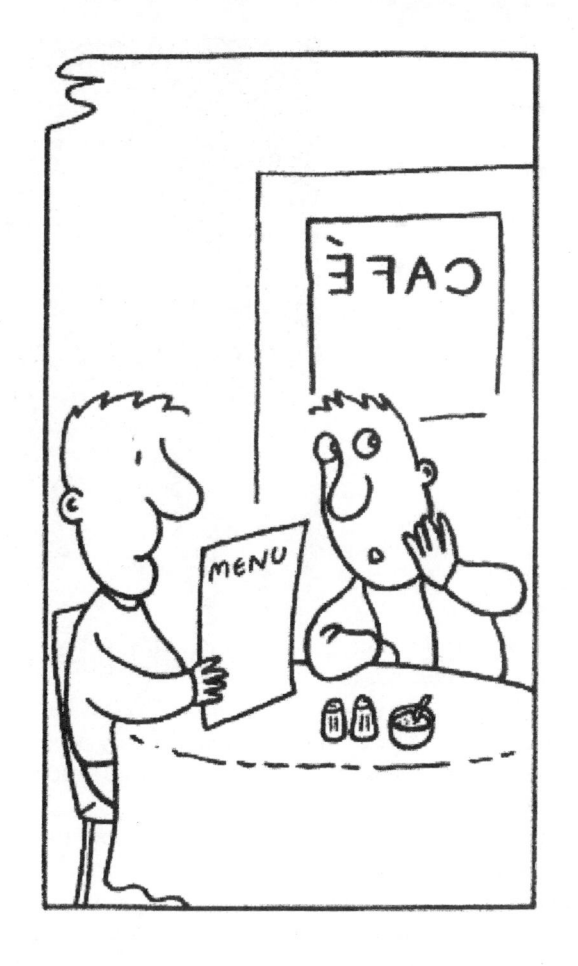

"First time I've been
able to enjoy pottering around
shops and museums without
feeling guilty about not being
up a fell……."

from The Kings. I agreed, but didn't think Pavarotti was available for bookings! Anyway, I digress. Several pints later an idea was formed – 'A Village Fair' with live music, street entertainment and craft stalls, a sort of Edinburgh Festival meets Petticoat Lane. Lots of fun, entertainment for everyone and above all a chance for local businesses to do something to attract those longed for and sorely missed visitors whilst enjoying a really fun packed day, a day we could all look forward to.

Planning this event has been a real roller coaster of experiences. Sitting at my desk trying to sort out which craft stall goes where. Keeping the fire-eaters and balloon modelling far enough apart, not to mention the awful moment when I realised that Tony Merrick's beloved pigeons would be flying above the village at about the same time as the clay pigeon shooting competition. You can imagine the picture of carnage that was forming in my mind. That aside, the hastily formed committee has without exception worked so hard and with such enthusiasm. A wonderful blend of like minded people, some from the Country Show Committee whose experience has been invaluable and others like myself, totally new to the organising events game. There have been many lessons learned along the way, (one poor sod can now quote word for word the latest Public Safety Act) and on a personal note, I really hope that the nights when I sit up in bed shouting 'bunting!' are at an end.

The National Trust have pulled out all the stops and taken on the job of organising a sports' day and kids fun day on our recreation field, although I did feel their plan to have Peter Rabbit abseiling from a helicopter was a little ambitious. The National Park heard our pleas of poverty and have generously agreed to donate all the village car parking fees taken on that day to our list of local good causes such as the Pre-school Playgroup. Hawkshead football club will become car park attendants for the day with some even planning on dressing up as highway robbers! And just when I thought I'd seen everything I came out of the Co-op and was met by a man riding through the village on a motorised toilet. 'It's for the Fair' he said. 'We're having a toilet race!' Of course we are. After all, this is Hawkshead, a delightful blend of community spirit and the completely bonkers.

So, what are my hopes for the day? Well, fine weather would be a real godsend. I think I've said enough 'Hail Marys' to earn us fine weather for the rest of the year! My greatest wish is that the shops, cafes and pubs have a really busy day and that visitors and locals enjoy the entertainment we've organised for them. Also, I hope that people will see that as devastating as foot and mouth has been, we are still here and trying desperately to create something positive out of a truly awful situation.

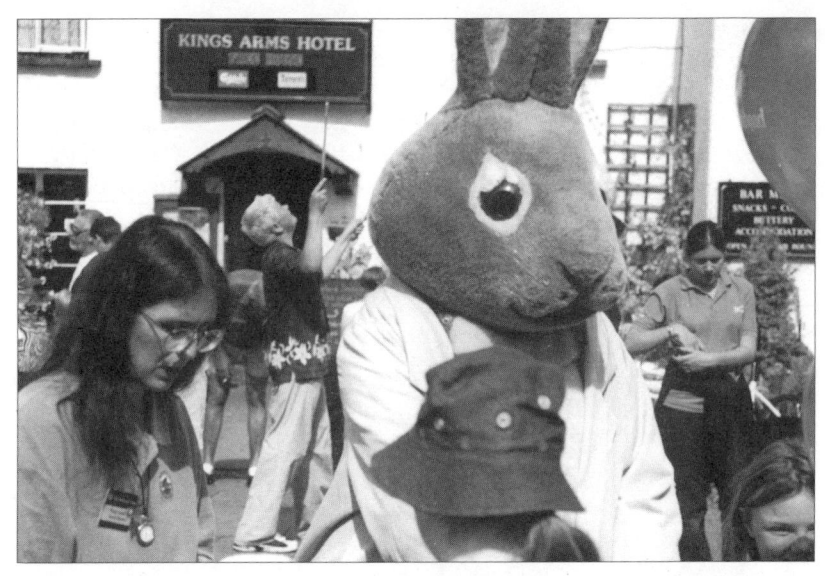

Peter Rabbit declines the invitation to abseil from a helicopter keeping his paws firmly on the ground, seen here soaking up the atmosphere at Hawkshead Village Fair

Thursday 23rd August.
The day after. Here again only this time I'm poised between complete exhaustion and absolute elation. Oh yes, and with a very slight hangover! I'm pleased to report that my many prayers were answered and the sun shone all day. Crowds of people came, so many, in fact, that I thought the rest of South Lakeland must have been deserted. There were so many highlights of the day it's hard to know which ones to mention. The craft and home produce competition was a great success, although I had to laugh when Jackie, one of the organisers, came to me and said that the village postmistress was the only tart in the village - custard of course! The toilet race was....... bizarre, to say the least. And the entertainers kept everyone enchanted all day. We finished off with a superb, lively ceilidh in the market square. I have been both delighted and humbled by the huge effort made by many people. They have made our drink induced ramblings into a glorious reality. I think I can say that without exception everyone had a wonderful day when our troubles and worries were put to the back of our minds. The mood now is one of optimism and hope.

Holly – The Redundant Collie

Holly, a four year old border collie, has been in full time employment at Swaledale Watch Farm, Whelpo since early pup-hood. The foot and mouth outbreak of 2001 left her unemployed and exceedingly bored. Unable to find work with MAFF (later DEFRA) like many others in her situation, Holly had to look for new ways to keep herself busy.

I was having the time of my life. It was lambing time. I was that bit older and I was trusted to work with the newly-born lambs this year. We had long days, my master and I, but all was going so well, we were both in our element.

Then one day the sheep all disappeared in huge lorries. I couldn't understand it. Everyone was crying. Did I do something wrong? What happened?

The long boring days became long boring weeks. I never thought I would have a problem with my weight, but I have to admit, I am a little tubbier than I should be. Yes, we started going for walks, still do. I laid around in the sunshine, still do. But still no sheep. I tried to think of things to do and ways to help. I thought they might want me to round up the miniature horses, but honestly, they're so stupid they wouldn't be driven. I tried everything: barking, stalking, running back and forth, but no, they didn't play the game at all. Then I thought about the hens. Same again. They wouldn't do as I

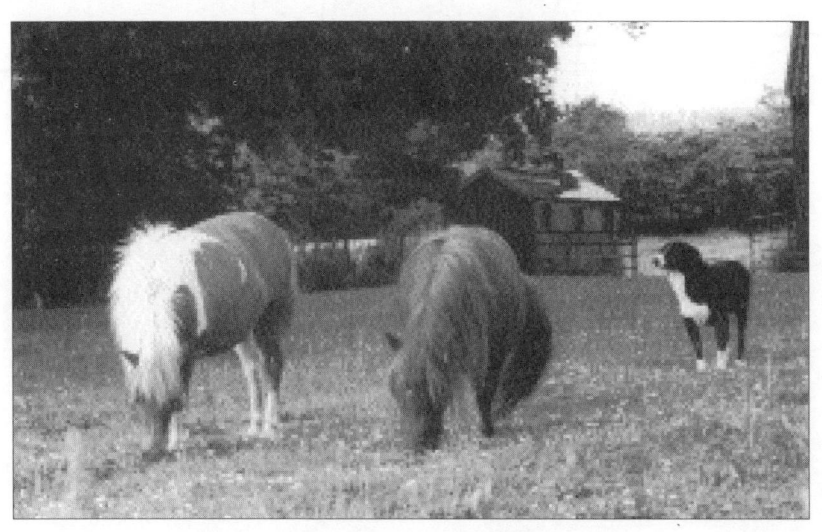

You can lead a collie to ponies..........!

wanted at all. I had heard quite a lot of my collie friends had been given ducks to round up and they thoroughly enjoyed that. Me! I just get hens who only want to scratch around and have dust-baths.

Then I discovered a real novel way to use up all my boundless energy. The master's wife does B & B. Guess what? These mainly city people who come to stay think it is hilarious when I help show them around. I can get them to the front door in a few general and gentle manoeuvres and it is really nice when the mistress opens the door and everyone is smiling – and all because I am only doing my job. Honestly, these horses, hens and people make sheep seem such intelligent creatures.

So here I am, longing to be back with my beloved sheep and having to do with rounding up people in the meantime. Roll on restocking.

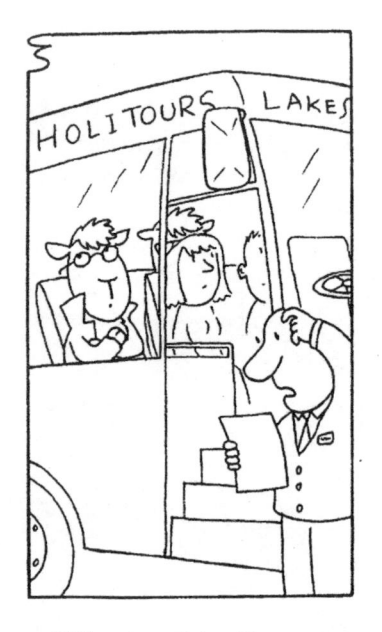

"That's odd - I've got more visitors leaving the Lakes than I had when I came here ......"

Mary Forster

Mary Forster farms at Weary Hall Style at Mealsgate near Wigton along with her husband and son. They lost more than 400 dairy cows and beef cattle, as well as 350 sheep to foot and mouth.

Today is the 1st of August. We have been officially signed off as 'clean' after a seemingly endless disinfecting process. It's hard to believe what was involved in getting our farm past the inspectors. This is what happened.

We were confirmed with foot and mouth on Thursday the 22nd of March. Our stock was slaughtered and after a long wait the farm was finally cleared of our animals so we could start to do something. My husband, son and worker (Tony, Ian and Michael) began with the cleaning process. All the muck had to be cleared from the sheds before we could begin with the pressure washers. Busying ourselves was a good way to get rid of the memories of the last fortnight. After 3 weeks the farm had had its usual spring clean only slightly earlier than normal, although there is nothing normal about this year. Now we thought we would sit back and leave it to the contractors to cleanse, disinfect, de-grease etc. How wrong we were! Our team arrived. Six Scousers, along with a Portakabin, Portaloo, dirty water tanks, tractors, cherry pickers and pressure washers. Once again, as with slaughter day, our farm had been taken over. Within a week we were on good terms with these strangers who were systematically taking our farmstead to pieces. They were in charge, we were just working along side them. For the first time in our lives we were not in charge of decision making on the farm. Even though they were a good bunch we longed for the day when our farmyard would be ours again. I got busy baking for them and each day they would bring me an empty tin back for more cakes. Small gestures were much appreciated and they looked forward to coffee time.

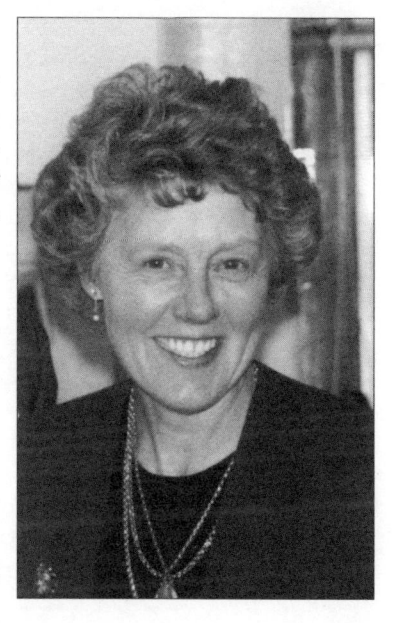

After 7 weeks of intensive activity when every nook and cranny had every spec of dirt removed it was time for the team to move on. We thought we would be able to get back to looking after the farm and managing the grassland which the cows and sheep would normally have done for us. However the men from the ministry had other ideas. The next phase of the cleansing was slurry removal. As usual with MAFF there were lots of false starts as to what was going to happen. Eventually an enormous machine arrived which would mix the slurry with lime and inject it into the ground. This was followed by another team of men who were to clean the slurry pits. Equipped with breathing apparatus and lifelines they were lowered into the pits with their high pressure hoses to clean up. Every day there were different faces around, and again we felt trapped in our own surroundings: people were coming and going oblivious to our existence, even thought they were on our farm. The next team to arrive was the milking parlour team which set about taking the milking equipment to pieces and disinfecting it. A place which should have been bustling with cows became an empty shell with all the parts stored in plastic bags in a corner.

At last we thought the end was in sight, but things are not that simple when you're working with MAFF. Our first inspection day arrived, now we'll get our lives back. We thought we were cleaner than clean – the concrete was shining, not a cobweb in sight, even the swallows had clean rafters to nest in. The Animal Health Officer arrived with hammer and knife, a tap on a gate here, a scrape with the knife there. No, it wasn't good enough. Out came the pressure washers again, this time manned by ourselves. The size of the list of jobs left to do, it felt like we were starting from scratch again. Slats to be pressure washed again and gates to be scrubbed with steel wool to remove any trace of debris. The old stone buildings which have been white washed for scores of years were not up to standard. Holes in walls had to be filled in with cement; in fact if you saw a crack anywhere, fill it in. Cobbles on the stable floor which were so much part of the character of the old buildings had to be cemented over to get rid of the invisible enemy. By this time the summer had nearly disappeared. Spring never happened. We were unaware of the seasons, no lambs to see, no excited cattle getting turned out onto fresh grass. Our awareness of the seasons had been lost in the frenzy of the clean up.

Once again we were anticipating the visit of the Animal Health Officer, this time, surely everything would be to the required standard.

Probably for the first time in months we started to look forward. For so long we had so many people about, but they were all strangers, now at last after almost four months we felt it was safe to see our family again. There were many emotional reunions during this time, some with friends who were in the same position as ourselves, others who still had their animals but who were also under enormous pressure.

For four months all our thoughts were consumed with cleansing and disinfection and complying with regulations which MAFF had imposed upon us. At last we felt we could look a little to the future, still not sure when we would be allowed to farm again, our thoughts turned to cows, semen catalogues, milk prices, price of quota, milk purchasers,...... all the things which had had little meaning in our lives over the past months.

The Animal Health Officer arrived and slowly made his way around all the buildings with a magnifying glass! Really. What seemed like an age later he came to tell us that we were clean and that our FM7 would be signed. No more pressure washers but still plenty of work, everything which was taken apart will have to be put together again - the milking parlour, the cow mats, cubicles, feed barriers all to be put back into working order.

So much for a quiet summer. We've never been so busy and still a long way to go before the place is alive with the smells and sounds of animals again.

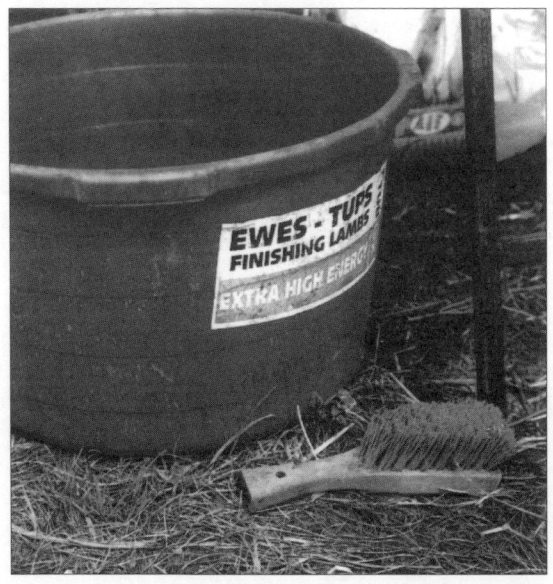

Photo: John Darwell

John Graham

John Graham farms beef cattle at Kirkbampton near Carlisle. His farm is just a few miles from the mass burial and slaughter site at Great Orton Airfield. His stock didn't contract foot and mouth disease but the regulations and restrictions that accompanied the outbreak made farming almost impossible for those who were left.

Kirkbampton Farm
Kirkbampton
Carlisle
CA5 6JB.

Dear Mr Hayward   1-6-2001.

    I do hope you have time to read this letter, during this difficult and hectic time in your department. Although I know, I'm only one of many hundreds of local people suffering during this horrible situation we've all found ourselves in. I'm hoping I can appeal to you personally to ease the pressure I'm now under.

    You will see from my address I live in Kirkbampton. Our Parish has 22 farms. Only 3 now survive. With a lot of luck, admittedly, but also a lot of hard work and care our farm is one of these 3.

    Since March 8th I have been in a D Zone. Since March 10th F&M has been on my doorstep. The daily feeding and the frequent inspections have been attended to with trepidation. As spring arrived and the need to leave the farmyard to complete seasonal field work was forced upon me, this was approached with fear.

    During this time, like you, I have witnessed terrible scenes. I've watched, from my bedroom window, the flames of the funeral pyre dance around the carcasses of my neighbours animals. Friends of over 40 years who live directly opposite. I listened to the sickening regularity of the efficiency of the humane killers at my neighbours alongside me. Our buildings are only 14 yards apart. I smelled the stench of death from the endless procession of Snowie wagons.

    I have now lived with F&M for 12 weeks but only now do I feel a victim. Though thankfully restrictions are relaxing you don't know how frustrating it is to have to ring numbers endlessly before getting information. Moving cattle to summer grazing. Normally a swift enjoyable task becomes an endurance event. The selling of fat cattle. A time to reap the financial rewards of months of hard work has become nothing more than a painful relief, the cost of feeding housed cattle is greater than their liveweight gain. Worst of all are these endless surveilance checks. Do MAFF not trust me? I have no milk cows, no pedigree breeding cattle why would I hide anything! Why do other farmers not have checks?

Living, as I do, within 3km of Great Orton burial site I hear constant rumours. The worst one being that MAFF are so frightened of the monster they've create that they want a 3km zone around the site free of all animals. Last week the fourth last survivor in the Parish lost his animals. Taken on suspicion of F&M. Are you taking us out one by one? Are these constant surveilance visits waiting for a chance to get me on suspicion of F&M. Am I waiting on death row? I'm sure a criminal committed of the most heinous crim wouldn't be kept under the mental pressure I'm now feelin

Would it be possible to stop these visits? If not would it be possible to have my cattle blood tested, by my own vets and visits stopped, assuming they were negative. If surveilance visits are to continue could I be given a time sheet and allowed to charge MAFF for the time I spend with the vets. I would wish to backdate this to early May when I was first checked.

I look forward to an early reply to my problems.

yours sincerely

JJ Graham.

This is a copy of a letter John sent to Andrew Hayward, MAFF and later DEFRA's Head of Veterinary Operations in Carlisle. Mr Hayward replied by return of post.

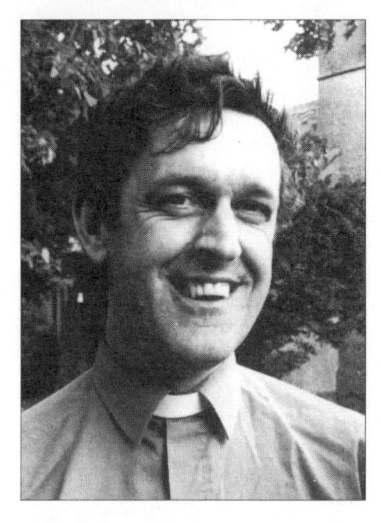

David Wood

David Wood has spent the past six years as Priest-in-Charge of the parishes of Asby, Bolton and Crosby Ravensworth, which made up part of the so-called 'Penrith Spur'. The 'Spur' escaped relatively unscathed in the early days of the foot and mouth outbreak only to find almost all of its livestock devoured by the virus in July and August, a tragedy largely ignored by the national press.

For some twelve years, earlier in my life, I was a herdsman on dairy farms in north Lancashire and I have never lost my love of the countryside and its people. I grew up in the Ullswater valley so the opportunity for ministry just a few miles away was welcome.

When the first news of foot and mouth broke back in February it was more than just another piece of news. It was something that made the heart miss a beat because of its potential effects, effects which have been all too clearly seen and felt here in these parishes in the last few weeks.

It is now mid August. Sandwiched as we are between the Lake District, the Pennines and the Yorkshire Dales, this is not a big tourist area and there is little scope for diversification there. The roads are even quieter than normal. It feels that we are alone, that no one wants to know. The belated setting-up of major disinfection points on the edge of this area only makes things worse. Now we are infectious, not just suffering from a disease. Agriculture remains the mainstay of the community yet it has been rocked to its very roots. The fields are empty and the fells are quiet. There are only a handful of farms in this area with any stock left. Thistles and thin wispy grass grows on pasture as well as the open fell. How much we take for granted! A casual passer-by would probably not appreciate much more than that, and why should they? The surface problem, of no stock, is only too evident; it is the long-term effects that are far more worrying. This is a community in shock, which feels forgotten, ignored and isolated. The Breacon Beacons lost large numbers of stock one recent weekend; we lost three times that number at the same time and the national press never noticed. The local press have done a good job though.

> **DEFRA**
> Department for
> Environment,
> Food & Rural Affairs
>
> Thank you for calling in to have your vehicle cleansed and disinfected. This is an important part in the effort to stop the spread of the Foot & Mouth Virus
>
> *Many Thanks*

This is a community with suddenly almost no income and with few resources other than the natural resilience of its people. The tragedy that has overtaken it beggars belief. Other communities further north who suffered equally badly back in March and April can perhaps now begin to look forward, but not this one, not yet. We have a winter to face, a winter with little to do and, perhaps more of a problem, little incentive to do anything. Indeed, why bother when ultimately your livelihood is in the hands of people who appear to have made little effort to get to grips with a problem or who have little concept of the complex relationships between people, land and animals. There are a few farms grimly clinging on to livestock. Perhaps more than any, they are the forgotten ones. The one dairy farm left in this parish is in a ravine. It cannot be seen from the road, and they cannot see anything else.

Inevitably in this 'pressure-cooker' kind of existence we have lived under, personal relationships begin to strain and habits begin to change. One person tends to work more regular hours, with weekends off; will milking cows on a dark morning be easy to go back to? Another finds that other things are now possible. A third finds that his business, which has only been ticking over before this is suddenly in demand.

We no longer have funeral pyres standing as beacons so that all can see where this unseen enemy has hit. Just rows of trucks clogging narrow lanes. Things just disappear. The cows at Crosby Hall right behind our house went in for milking one afternoon and never came out again, at least, not walking.

And yet, and yet. As so often happens, in the midst of all this unwarranted destruction lies the seed of new life, of renewal. At the moment it is probably unrecognised as new by those most caught up in events, but I am sure they are there. Time after time my thoughts go to the Old Testament prophet Habakkuk, who recognises that in spite of disaster, God is still God.

He writes, 'Even though the fig trees have no blossoms, and there are no grapes on the vine; even though the olive crop fails, and the fields lie empty and barren; even though the flocks die in the fields, and the cattle barns are empty, yet I will rejoice in the Lord! I will be joyful in the God of my salvation.'

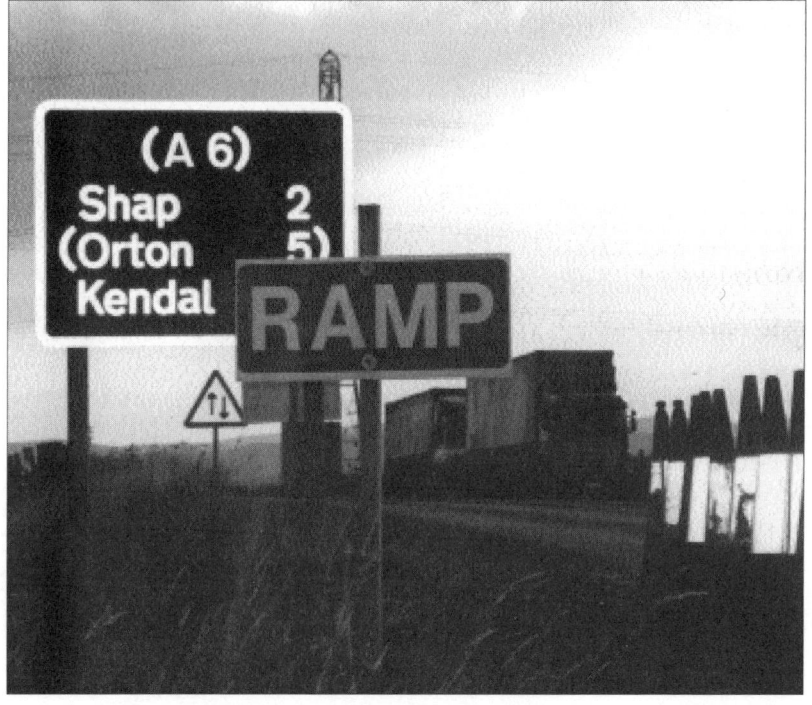

Photo: Caz Graham

Nick Green

Nick Green is an outdoor activities instructor. When foot and mouth broke out he was unable to do his normal work and found himself more and more affected by the ghastly images he found all around him at his home in Long Marton, between Penrith and Appleby. Desperate to contribute to the fight against the disease he helped set up the 'Heart of Cumbria' organisation.

Silent spring, silent summer – silent autumn?

A lamb cowers by the side of the road shivering, isolated from its mother and the flock. Men are shouting across the moor, dogs are barking and I hear the revving of several quad bikes. Two thousand ewes and their lambs are being gathered from Orton Scar. They are to be slaughtered here today. The slaughter men await their arrival, chatting in the morning sun and eating the delights found in their bait boxes. The collies work well, efficiently and enthusiastically. The Snowie detox lorries are in position and some of the ewes are already caged, unaware of their impending fate.

This is August 2001, the seventh month of the foot and mouth crisis and the killing continues with no end in sight. These are hefted flocks, sheep that have grazed these moors for hundreds of years. Irreplaceable stock and, unbelievably, healthy. Over the past few months I have witnessed many other scenes similar to this and it still sickens me. One of the most horrific was a couple of miles from my home. A large pile of dead ewes lay by the side of the road. Hanging from the rear of many of these ewes were aborted lambs. No words can describe such scenes.

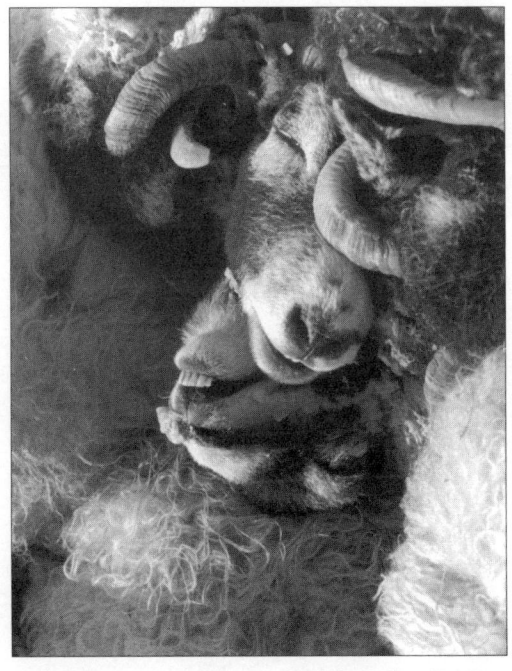

Photo: Nick Green

When the BBC announced in late February that foot and mouth had been discovered in Northumberland, I turned to my wife Helen and we agreed that this was likely to be very serious. We listened intently to every news report. Gradually the scale of the impending disaster unravelled.

Many tragic stories were told and rumours were rife: farmers awakening to the bellowing of cattle that had survived the cull, surrounded by the carcasses of the rest of their herd. Sheepdogs being killed after the gather - did this really happen? Lambs having their throats cut, and other culls being badly botched. Each one of these reports and rumours must have had a devastating effect on all who heard them, including me.

It was against this background that I became uneasy. There was something amiss here. How could I find out more? I turned to the Internet. I studied web sites such as Peter Kindersleigh's 'Sheep Drove', Jane Barribal's 'Farm Talking' and many more. There was plenty of time for all this research because I had now lost all my work. I am a freelance outdoor activities instructor and I had been informed that the contract I was to be awarded with a local Outdoor Education Centre was not to be honoured. It was inevitable as there were currently no courses being run in the centre. Foot and mouth was gripping all areas of rural life.

I spent the next few months studying every aspect of the disease. I made contact with other like-minded individuals not only within the UK but around the world. I needed to do more! But what? I spoke several times on BBC Radio Cumbria and wrote many letters to Government officials and others but there had to be something else I could do to help the situation. I attended an open meeting in Skipton. There the locals appeared to be far more outspoken and angry than here in Cumbria. They invited me to speak. I did so but very reluctantly. I spoke from the heart. They applauded and I was invited to a second meeting. I appeared on Channel 4 in June and in early July my friend Elaine Commander and I decided it was about time we had our own 'open meeting' here in Cumbria. It was held at Penrith Rugby Club and about 400 people turned out for it. Dr Ruth Watkins, a virologist and sheep farmer spoke about vaccination, Dr Richard North talked about the complex political component of the disease and Tom Lowther spoke passionately about the effects this tragedy had had on farming. I chaired the meeting, one of the hardest things I have ever done, but also one of the most rewarding. It was here that we decided to launch 'Heart of Cumbria'. The 'Hearts of Britain' organisation has been established to represent everyone who lives, works and has an interest in the countryside and 'Heart of Cumbria' is a way of making our voice heard, here in this county.

As the weeks merge into months I continue to try to 'do my bit'. I went on the demonstration in London organised by David Hanley of Farmers for Action and I was privileged to be allowed to deliver to 10 Downing Street, the thousands of signatures we had collected to petition the Prime Minister for a Public Inquiry. I felt privileged to represent this county. 'Heart of Cumbria' is expanding rapidly and helping to get it up and running is taking every spare minute!

It is now late August and there is no end in sight to this tragedy. The crisis has dominated my life for the last 6 months. Work colleagues tell me I have changed drastically. But then hasn't everything? Will this county ever return to normality? Yes, I have to hope so and I think it will. I'll continue to help with 'Heart of Cumbria' and from time to time I'll be outspoken on the radio or in my letters to the press. I am passionate about this county, its farming community and country life. At present it is decimated but I intend to fight to win it back and there are many others who feel just as strongly and will lend a hand. In the years to come I hope I'll be able to look back and know that I did my bit. It may have been a small effort but 'big trees from little acorns grow'!

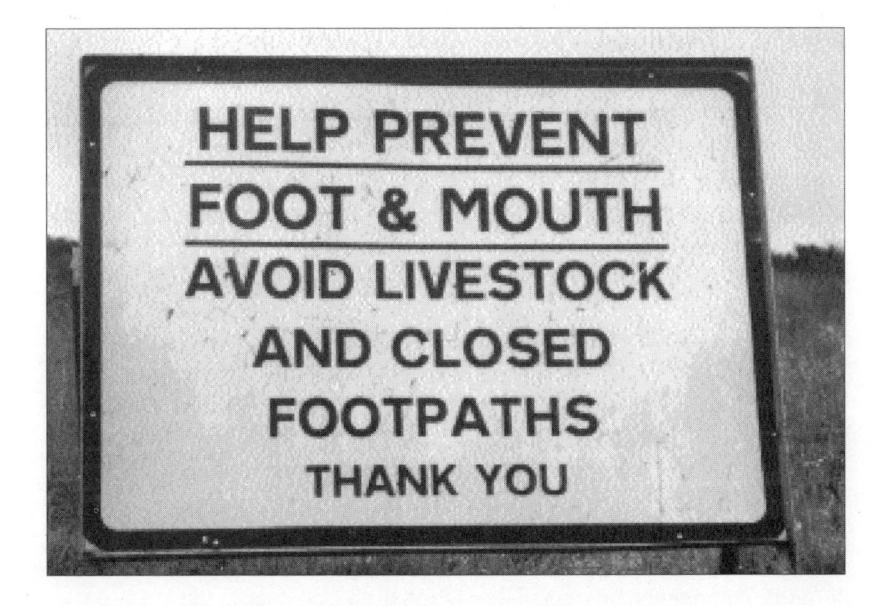

Andrew Humphries

Andrew Humphries is a well known figure in Cumbrian agricultural circles. He spent thirty years as teacher and mentor for new generations of farmers at Newton Rigg College near Penrith. He sits on the government Task Force for the Hills, and is a key player in Cumbria Farm Link, a business and environmental advisory service for farmers. During the foot and mouth outbreak Andrew, amongst other things, looked after a help-line on behalf of the Council for Agriculture and Rural Life (CARL) which is a Churches Together organisation.

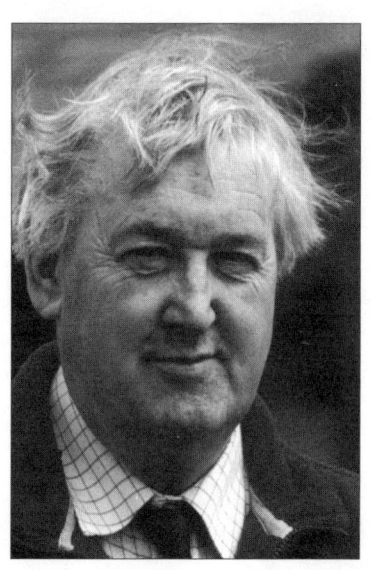

Photo: Farm Stock Photography

**'There was a Door to which I found no Key:
There was a Veil past which I could not see'**
Edward Fitzgerald

As I write at the end of August it seems that rural communities have struggled desperately to see beyond Edward Fitzgerald's veil, to find some small certainties in a world that seems increasingly uncertain. Who, amongst the rural communities of Cumbria and others touched by the epidemic, has not felt that depth of isolation in some measure?

Remarkably, prior to foot and mouth, many would have seen the rural churches as largely irrelevant and in decline, yet the implied question 'who is my neighbour' was answered without debate by ministers and people. One morning in early June my phone rang and the voice of a farmer's wife said,'our lovely vicar says I should ring you'. This was one of over 2000 such calls to our CARL help-line. The church's unique presence in each and every community presented a challenge and an opportunity which has brought hope where despair threatened to overwhelm.

Networks appeared almost as a natural consequence of need, vital to bring some confidence, purpose and practicality in our responses. Yet for the farming community, marginalised, isolated and confused, the very act of listening and trying to understand has seemed so important. So much in the national media seemed alien and made me angry; particularly the pictures that were being painted of farming people which conflict with experience and reality. Like many others I turned to the local radio and press which showed sensitivities which supported rather than damaged.

At the low point I looked from my window across to the northern fells through the smoke of numerous fires to the emptiness of a deserted landscape, resembling a beautiful stage set without the dynamic of actors or dialogue. So many of the calls were not only about foot and mouth; they concerned situations in which the epidemic overwhelmed the ability to cope with existing family crises and economic collapse. I still cannot quite grasp how some individuals and families survived the circumstances which perversely combined.

Babies were born and could not be shared with families, people died and could not be laid to rest in their own burial ground, children and students were separated from parents or from education. Employment off-farm was lost or sacrificed in the interests of bio-security and concern for neighbours.

Oliver Goldsmith wrote on hope in The Captivity: 'Hope like the gleaming taper's light, Adorns and cheers our way, And still as darker grows the night, Emits a brighter ray.' I have seen that 'gleaming taper's light' contrasted with all that is dark. The phone calls from people more concerned for others: the aunt concerned for her niece, followed in a few days by the niece ringing about her aunt. Separated and isolated by 30 miles yet together as members of a united family. At something of a low point I received a call from a fell farming family near Keswick. Speaking to each in turn we shared thoughts. Then I asked how I could help. 'You misunderstand' came the gentle reply, 'we were concerned about you!'

One of the major roles of the help-line I've been working on has been to link people with the funds available to help with disruption caused by foot and mouth. The Royal Agricultural Benevolent Institution and The Addington Fund at Stoneleigh have worked ceaselessly and selflessly to do what they can to ease the situation. Between two and three thousand families have received direct assistance. Many of the Addington grants were used to relieve animal welfare problems. A fodder merchant with whom I had many conversations performed minor miracles as a local Red Cross service.

Individual responses to need have perhaps inspired me more than I can easily express. Again, they are Goldsmith's 'gleaming taper's light'. I received a letter from a vet concerned at the situation on the farm that he had visited for MAFF. He asked that I receive a cheque for his fees for the two days work and that I send an anonymous cheque for that amount to the family. A farming family returned a cheque which had been sent from the

Addington Fund. They had in the meantime received money from a relative and wished the Addington money to be sent to someone 'in greater need'.

The support was not confined to those within the rural community and I took heart from the many letters and gifts from urban neighbours. An anonymous donation from Yorkshire was accompanied by a note, 'Our hearts go out to the farmers and their families - from two walkers who love and respect the countryside.' Bearing the hallmark of the widow's mite, a note accompanied a small cheque from Cheshire. 'May God add his blessings to this small donation, as he blessed the loaves and fishes.'

In our own parishes farming families received a card from the churches. The illustration used was the cross of nails, a symbol of hope made by a priest from three iron nails which fell from the blazing timbers of the roof of Coventry Cathedral during the second world war, a symbol of hope and resurrection. Six months into the epidemic with Cumbria fading from the national media and the concerns of government my spirits were lifted through a generous gift from the Mothers' Union in Coventry. How poignant that an urban community which itself had risen from the ashes of war should offer their support and concerns for this distant corner of rural England.

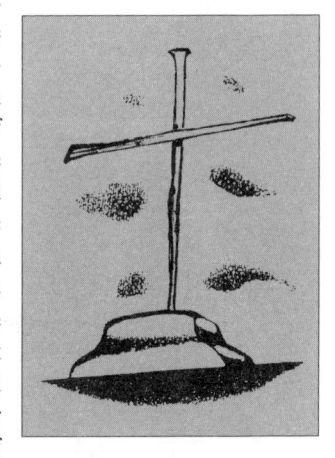

For some the pain is still acute, for others it may still be to come, yet vitally, people are looking forward and hoping for leadership that will enable them to rebuild. The way is not yet clear, neither will it be easy.

My hope is that it will be an integrated partnership. Just as working together has been a positive outcome of the crisis, it is self-evident that partnership is the only way forward, but with the focus on self-help and bringing together the whole community of Cumbria.

Wendell Berry the American Farmer-Poet wrote:-

'One resurrected community would be more convincing and more encouraging than all the government programmes of the past 50 years - but to be authentic, a true encouragement and a true beginning, this would have to be a resurrection accomplished mainly by the community itself.'

Pamela Brough

Pamela Brough is an Ulverston-based writer. For many years she farmed, wrote and broadcast from her small hill farm near the moorland village of Flash, in the Peak District.

My own farm is small, and I manage it from a distance, but with the first confirmed cases of foot and mouth, leaflets and letters from MAFF started to arrive. During conversations between myself, my local MAFF officer, family and neighbours in farming, I found myself making notes. When Carole Hamby from Kendal Windows on Art asked if I would take part in a cultural documentation of the effects of foot and mouth on farmers and others here in Cumbria, the notes became a series of scribed encounters. People were free to say what they felt, what they feared, what they suspected. My job was to write down exactly what they said. The outcome is a collection of voices which will become part of the National Farming Documentation programme, testimony to a crisis and, hopefully, a vehicle for discussion and change.

People were determined not to be sentimental. Nevertheless, the reality of mass death in buildings, yard or field needs recognition. All the statements about dead animals being the end product of livestock farming have been made by now, and no one really knows where to go with the facts.

It's part of a cycle, I was told by one person. She was quoting a slaughter man. He, too, was finding it hard to cope with the mass killing. He talked of having standards, of respecting the animals, giving them a decent death. The one-fell-swoop of a cull is something else. There is anger, despair, anguish. People come to kill all your stock. You don't want them there, but they turn out to be good people, kind, supportive. You can't hate them for what they are doing. But everything takes place against a conflict of advice, instruction, and policies from above. Something feels wrong. There's suspicion. What's really going on? Meanwhile, the images projected by people whose job is to have opinions, seem to come from another planet. In the end, you have to override the blame, the scandal mongering, the few sharp reminders that whatever the system, someone will try to take advantage of it. Listen instead to the ones whose determination to rebuild their empty farms is based on a whole chapter of grief and despair. A farmer from Carlisle told me, 'We have to use this as a way to improve on things – from farm practice, to markets, to supermarkets, to our relationship with customers who buy what we produce. We're listening; talk to us, tell us what you want us to do and we'll do it'. There's a big debate, waiting to happen.

Elegy

We don't need an interpreter:
what's true for one of you
another takes as challenge –
you shred our lives into
pieces of argument.

Let us tell our own tale:
how we came to this hill.
became part of it, like bed-rock,
mixing our dirt
with dust of hoof and horn,
hair and hide,
skin, bone, wool.

Connecting only where we touched –
what we walked on,
what we worked with.
Not worldly-wise, but strong.

The coffin lid slides shut.
Beneath it, put in photographs.

Here's our Jane with Mrs Wilson –
the sheep who came and went
through the open farmhouse door,
who could have had hay, straw,
a field, an orchard,
company of cows, pigs, chickens – even her own kind –
who settled for
a slot between TV and bookcase,
wedging herself in tight,
fleece displacing rows of classic prose,
conversationally baa-ing back at the telly.

Put in the urge to save
lives, landing on our doorstep
the inadequate humans,
trying to be parent birds
to a trio of dying swallows -
Why don't they eat?
What is their expectation?
How can we deliver it?

Put in our ingenuity -
the cut-out shadow-bird,
shape, enough; size, enough
to trip the wire of their
unavoidable bird-nature -
and set them beaks a-gape,
taking in flies.

Put in the generosity of hours;
of time tuned to a dandelion clock -
slow, and slow - then
sudden quick breath of harvest,
and Sweet! Sweet! -
of swallows,
skimming the sky.
Put in the joy of it -
before the world moved
from the end of the lane,
to the edge of the meadow,
to outside the window,
to into our house.

Close the lid gently
as you put us away.

Les Armstrong

Les Armstrong is the Chairman of the NFU's national Livestock Committee. He farms in the Eden Valley at Blunderfield, Kirkoswald. Les's own cattle were some of the first in the county to fall victim to foot and mouth and the moving account he gave on both radio and television of how it felt to lose his stock touched many people. His spring and summer were consumed in an endless stream of Ministerial visits, meetings and interviews with the media while representing Cumbrian farmers.

On approximately the 17th of February 2001 France announced it was considering a ban on UK lamb, because of doubts over scrapie in sheep. On the 19th of February the EU Commission announced new proposals on the Beef Support System to address problems caused by the discovery of BSE in several other EU countries. Both of these measures would have been damaging to UK farmers so on the 20th of February I went to Brussels with Ben Gill and others to express our concerns. When we arrived in the Brussels office we heard that foot and mouth disease had been discovered in Essex, but in our meeting with Commission officials we concentrated on the first two points as foot and mouth disease was a little local problem which would be dealt with and stamped out. How wrong we were! Even when it was discovered around Longtown we still thought everything would be quickly traced and slaughtered – it had to be: I had cancelled our foot and mouth insurance policy the year before! Never in our wildest thoughts did we think it would arrive at Blunderfield, but as we now know, foot and mouth shows no discretion. I will remember forever walking past our cubicle sheds and Martin shouting 'Dad, you'd better come in here. We've got it.'

What happened next has been well recorded and like hundreds of families, including many who are not directly involved in farming, we have gone through five months of mixed emotions. It is only now, as we get the farm ready for restocking, that we are beginning to realise the effect this disease has had on our farm. After a week or two when we got used to the eerie silence, we had to start thinking about what we were going to do. Obviously the buildings were going to stand empty until the disease was cleaned out, but what to do with the land was the big problem. It would have been very easy just to close the gates and forget about it, but after years of improving the farm and creating a well managed landscape, we were not prepared to let it turn into a wilderness. Like many others farmers, we ploughed more land to grow grain and bought a machine to cut grass and keep the remaining pasture in good condition. However, it is ironic that the year we have no livestock has been very good for growing grass, so we have finished up cutting most of the fields for silage and hay, some of which we will not need this winter, as we will not restock with the same number of animals as before.

At the same time, many farms in other parts of the county have far too much stock because of movement restrictions and will not have been able to conserve enough crop for winter. There will need to be massive movements of livestock and crop to get back to some sort of normal farming procedures. It will be a slow process at first, but it needs to happen as quickly as possible. As I write this on August the 10th 2001, farmers who are still farming are finding life very difficult to cope with. They are working longer hours to look after the extra stock, recovering less money for stock they sell for slaughter because of the lack of a proper market, and suffering all the extra cost and social consequences of bio-security measures. On the other hand, many farmers like us are not starting as early in the morning, have no daily problems with livestock and are enjoying easy weekends. This is not the life we are used to and we need to get back to our proper job!

Of course we will get the disease 'under control' and we have to make sure that good comes out of evil. At the moment many people are talking about change without knowing exactly what they mean, but there will be change on our farm at least. We are making alterations now to accommodate a larger dairy herd and the emphasis will be on quality of life rather than quantity of production. I have no doubt that the whole process of moving what we produce down the food chain will be looked at, and if it leads to a system where we can get a reasonable return for our efforts, then all well and good.

We must also have a fair return for landscape management, from which the whole country benefits.

So it is time to be positive and learn lessons from this awful disaster, one of which must be an end to the myth that agriculture is not important. It may no longer be the main industry, but in a

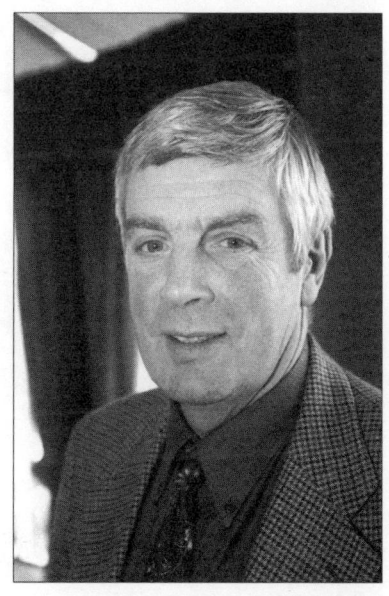

Photo: News & Star

county like Cumbria, it is the sledge that many other businesses slide on. First of all we need to see an end to the plague of foot and mouth, a proper inquiry to enable us to avoid it ever happening again and then acceptance of the important part agriculture plays in any rural economy. I know it is going to be difficult in the future persuading Government and the tax payer that farming will need continued support, but like any other industry the Government helps, it should not be a question of 'how much', but is it 'good value for money'. Winning this argument will be essential, not only for the countryside and the people who live in or visit it, but especially to create enthusiasm in the next generation of young farmers. At the moment we are bowed but not beaten!

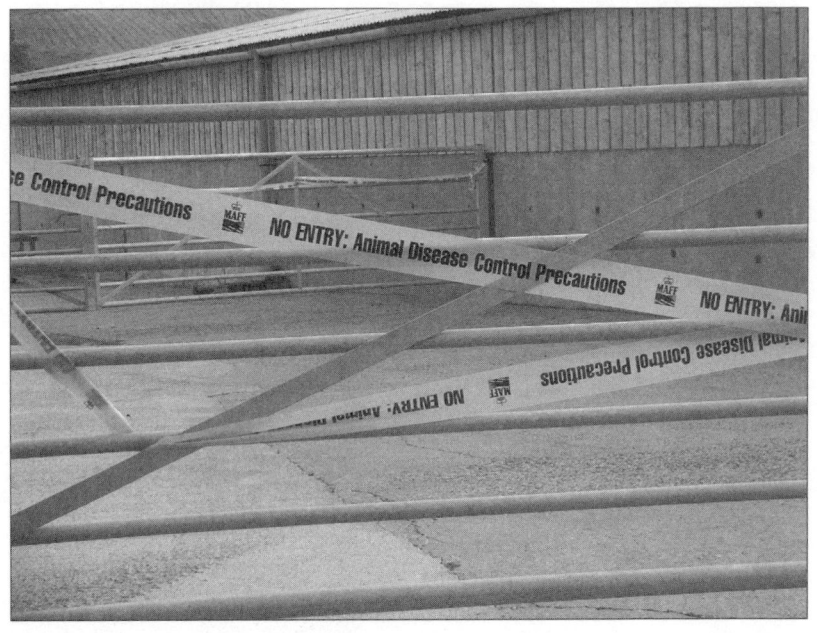

Photo: Rigby Jerram

Martin Lewes

Martin Lewes is the Kendal district journalist for BBC Radio Cumbria, and at the time the epidemic began was also producing and presenting the station's Farm and Countryside programme

Journalism, I once told a politician, is a game for voyeurs. She'd asked me whether I'd ever considered going into politics, say as a local councillor. I told her I preferred watching, asking questions, and telling people what I'd found out.

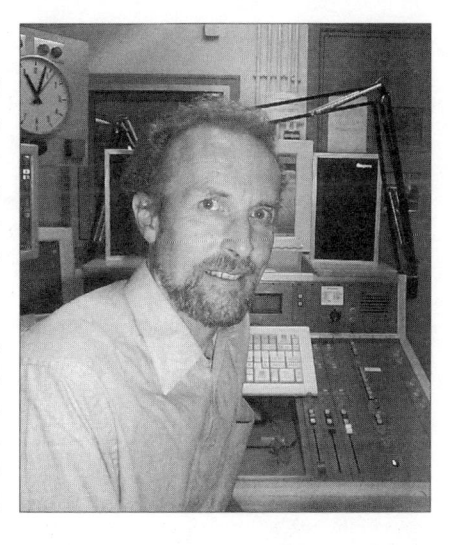

But there is of course more to it than that. Simply by being there, by asking questions and publicising the answers, journalists can change things. So looking back now over the four or five months since foot and mouth began its surge through Cumbria, it's only human to wonder whether we - I - did change anything. Should we have done? Could we - I - have done more to lessen the carnage the disease wrought across the infected farms, to reduce the number of animals slaughtered before their time, the despair of the farmers who didn't lose their own stock, but found their businesses ruined as normal marketing came to a halt, the distress of those who found the fields next to their homes a scene of infernal burning or of heaps of dead animals for days or weeks? Could we have lessened what soldiers call the collateral damage, on the tourism industry - put like that it sounds cold, but the pain of a couple who've spent years building up their bed and breakfast trade, only to spend weeks with empty rooms, watching their bank balances turn red, is no less that that of anyone else who finds what they thought the safe ground of their livelihoods beginning to shake and sink beneath their feet.

Part of my memory is that it seemed to come on like one of those tidal bores that sweep across Morecambe Bay when the time is right. The bore comes with the speed of a galloping horse, they say - but, watching, it seems small and slow at first in the distance, only piling into its full force and momentum as it gets closer. That misleading stateliness has cost the lives of walkers on the sands, swept away by what seems at first a ripple, only to become a towering surge of water when it's far too close to outrun.

So it was, from that dusk when I stood watching the flames take hold on a hundred-yard long pyre just outside Tirril, at the county's second infected farm, to when the whole of north Cumbria seemed to stink of the smell of burning hide. I said in my report that the fire would burn for days to consume a fine dairy herd and nine and a half thousand sheep. It burned for weeks, and within those weeks was only one of dozens, their smoke surging into the low winter clouds, the red glow patterning the countryside at night.

A week or two later I went into the animal health centre at Carlisle, to interview the top district vet, Andrew Hayward. The staff there had the red-ringed eyes of the deeply exhausted. I asked him whether he had enough people, enough resources generally. If he needed more, he replied, he could ask for them. I already knew he had the power, if he wished, to ask for military help – he hadn't yet done so, and that was his answer.

Shortly afterwards I was interviewing the farming minister, Joyce Quinn. Her boss, Nick Brown, had just said the epidemic – he didn't call it that – was under control. I suggested that this sounded from Cumbria like whistling in the wind. Down the line from the London studio came reassurance. Yes, she said, resources were stretched, but work was proceeding to identify the infected farms, to slaughter the animals there and dispose of the carcasses.

I told her that from here her organisation seemed overwhelmed, her staff exhausted. The minister replied calmly that should they need more people, more resources, they would be provided, that more staff were going in, that she was in contact with many people in Cumbria. She knew the situation in detail and was confident everything possible was being done.

When you interview a minister you have only a few minutes. I had other areas to cover, and I moved on.

But for me that interview hangs in the mind. Should I have hammered home the point? Should I have repeated the question, talked of the growing mounds of dead rotting stock in the fields, the days people were waiting even for a vet to come to see the stricken animals, never mind for the slaughter teams. It was to be at least another fortnight before first, the government's Chief Vet Jim Scudamore, then the fleets of army Land Rovers, the legendary Brigadier Alex Birtwistle, the extra vets and slaughter teams moved in to take the situation by the scruff of the neck. If I had driven the minister harder on the point, played Paxman and told her it looked like chaos here, over and again, would it have made a difference?

Later, after the soldiers and the rest of the cavalry arrived, it was the Prime Minister in a distant studio in London, my colleague Gordon Swindlehurst asking the questions. The first we agreed: 'Prime Minister, why did it take so long?'

Again, his answer was calm. At the start, he said, no one knew where the infection would be worst. It would've been easy but wrong, he said, to rush in resources to one place, only to find a new outbreak of disease in another. Now it was known how bad things were in Cumbria, no effort would be spared, whatever was needed would be supplied. There was – and it came out in spades when without warning, he visited Carlisle the following day – more than reassurance. People who were in the meeting at the Auctioneer came out walking on air, convinced battle was now fully joined and foot and mouth would soon be in retreat. They spoke of how Mr Blair, as each problem was mentioned, would turn to his civil servants and military staff, and order it dealt with. They also spoke of how the civil servants raised the difficulties, while the army, in the sturdy presence of Brigadier Birtwistle, simply made another note on his action list, but that's by the way.

I had a peculiarly semi-detached relation to the crisis. For most of the week FMD was simply a part of the news diet of my normal job as South Cumbria reporter - along with the council meetings, the industrial stories, and so on. The foot and mouth story around Kendal was farmers who couldn't move or sell their stock.

But as producer and presenter of our Farm and Countryside programme - normally a pleasant excuse for rambling around the countryside talking to interesting people - I was close to the heart of the station's coverage. I spent an increasing amount of time trying to make it what my managers called the 'must listen'. For me, this meant making sure we spoke to organ grinders, not monkeys - we had chief executives, directors, top politicians, people who could give answers as well as ask the right questions. I had a weekly date with the MAFF head of operations, Jane Brown for a recorded briefing – sometimes informative, sometimes anodyne. And at least a couple of days a week, I drove from Kendal to Carlisle. It was an instructive journey.

I would press on out of town up the A6 towards Shap past fields with sheep - and later in the year, lambs. Over the top on to the M6 and down towards Penrith, and the smell would come first. Then I would see the smoke, sometimes rising vertically into the air, sometimes rolling along the ground, and I wondered what it must be like to be downwind of such a thing. I watched for when the first pyre appeared as the disease moved south. Then I watched for when the fields became empty. Finally I would turn in past the Borderway Mart, which became a huge marshalling yard for trucks, coal, timber, the impedimenta of Brigadier Birtie and Jane Brown's battle. When you knew what was happening, it was hard to believe Kendal and Carlisle were in the same county.

We watched and reported as the troops and civil servants, the vets and slaughter teams, arrived in force. The pyres burned with new determination, fleets of trucks rumbled through, camouflaged Land Rovers buzzed around in convoys. First thousands, then tens of thousands of cattle, sheep, pigs and goats were tumbled into the flames and then, as that fell into disrepute, into the enormous trenches of Great Orton airfield. The resolution and dispatch with which the scientists' direction, kill infected stock within 24 hours, those on neighbouring farms within 48 hours, was put into action, impressed us – maybe even hypnotised us.

Because it was, however you might measure its success, a terrible purpose. I was asked by a Canadian radio station what the farmers went through. I described how some had found the first case among their dairy herd - in one, it was a calf whose tongue fell out when its mouth was opened, because the ulcers had eaten through the root. Farmers, I said, knew their stock was for a purpose, but some had wept when they spoke of the distress the disease caused their animals. I told of the wait for the vet, then for the slaughter teams, the hours inside the farmhouse while the rattle of captive-bolt guns echoed around the fields, then hours, maybe days more, while the stock burned. These animals, I said, might be destined for the slaughterhouse anyway, but they were dying before their time, and their bloodlines were often the result of generations of work by the same family. It was hard to tell that story.

And when that story is multiplied so many times, you have not single farms but whole springtime landscapes devoid of lambs and calves, whole communities enveloped in the smoke for days, a devastation of the little pattern of taking children to school, darts matches at the pub, Women's Institute meetings, trips to the shop or to friends which make up normal life – it was indeed a silent spring, and people did, as one councillor memorably said, seem to speak in whispers in the street.

And there were people who wanted to know, whether it really had to happen. There were continuing campaigns for vaccination, in spite of questions about its efficacy. We will never know whether a vaccine, swiftly distributed across the county's farms, could have slowed or even halted the epidemic. Many I spoke to, farmers and scientists, said the vaccine was not sufficiently reliable, that some inoculated animals remained infectious, that the anti-bodies vaccine would leave in the blood could not be told from those left by real infection, so masking the onward spread of the disease.

My own feeling at times was that the government had committed that cardinal sin of not knowing when it was in a hole, and failing to stop digging. Perhaps there was a moment when a switch of policies might have been possible.

But what is certain is what finally stopped that happening. On the continent farmers were offered vaccination. Then when the infection did stop, they were told the vaccinated animals would be slaughtered anyway. Not surprisingly, the lack of any promise not to do that in Britain meant that even when the government did offer the possibility, Cumbria's farmers swiftly rejected it. The rejection was swifter because only Cumbria's and Devon's farmers were being offered the vaccine. It would, they feared, label the county for years as the home of foot and mouth. In any case the vaccination would be for cattle, but not for sheep, when it was already known that the infection was spreading through sheep as much as cattle. There was too much confusion for anyone really to make a rational decision.

The darkest days did pass. The numbers of new cases dropped into single figures, and the chaos of the early days slipped quietly into the grim efficiency which meant rendering and burial could deal with the casualties. Those infernal pyres became an unrepeatable horror, a last resort. The signs of the disease, for most of the county, are the greener ungrazed fields, the emptiness of the hills where the numbers of sheep are at their lowest for years. Instead there is the hidden creep through the Penrith Spur, a few cases here and there every day or two. It could almost all be over.

But it isn't. At the time of writing, well over one million animals have been slaughtered in Cumbria alone. Perhaps half of Cumbria's farmers have no cattle or sheep. Many of the rest have lost some part of their stock. Even those that have lost nothing to the slaughter policy have found themselves struggling to feed animals for which there is still no real market. Their life is dominated by what's called bio-security. Every time they go on or off the public highway, the wheels of their tractors and cars must be washed and disinfected – the same for their footwear and, regularly, their clothes. They live, they'll tell you, on a knife edge, never knowing whether they'll go out to check the stock one day and find the symptoms - or, maybe worse, have a visit from the ministry vet to say that in some way they've had a dangerous contact with an infected farm and healthy or not, the animals must go. It's a knife-edge so sharp, they say, that it's almost a relief to fall off.

And the disease flickers on, bursting out here and there in small groups of farms - they seem small, but because neighbouring farms are, as they say, 'slaughtered out' as well, each of these sparks leaves another hamlet in silence. There is now for the farmers little hope of restocking this autumn, so they face the winter in idleness and uncertainty - long dark nights which, for one country clergyman I spoke to, threatened a yet deeper despair.

And we have - in economic terms, far more importantly - a tourism industry wondering whether enough visitors will come, leaving enough money behind to see those dozens of little businesses, guest houses, gift shops and cafes, through the winter. By the time you read this many people will have been invited to speak with their bank managers. Depending on how well they survived, some will be propped up through the low season, others will have been told that it would be better to give up now.

The inquests, of course, are yet to come. Journalists are taught that news can be broken down into the Ws - who, what, where, when and why, with why being the hardest to establish and usually the most interesting. The wilder end has already cost us hours. Is it true that infected parts of sheep have been found thrown into fields? Were orders really placed for huge quantities of railway sleepers and coal, weeks before the first disease? Was the National Farmers' Union really in cahoots with the government to wipe out tranches of small farmers and their stock, to bring subsidy payments under control and more order to over supplied markets? Even those rumours which can easily be followed have ended in a welter of 'I heard it from a cousin who overheard someone say in a pub that they'd been told it by someone who knew.....' We'll keep looking, but don't hold your breath. I suspect much of the truth will not come out for at least the thirty years for which Cabinet papers are kept from the public. Then it will be history, and will only become news if the truth is truly shocking. Even then, with those most deeply involved retired or dead, or at the very least no longer in government office, it'll be a one-day wonder. Reporting the truth then will make no difference now.

NO ENTRY: Animal Disease Control Precautions